SIRT FOOD DIET

MEAL PLAN:

A BEGINNERS GUIDE TO THE SIRT FOOD
DIET, TO ACTIVATE YOUR SKINNY GENE
AND BURN FAT WHILE EATING. WITH LOTS
OF HEALTHY RECIPES

Megan Parker

Table Of Contents

Introduction

S tarting the Sirtfood diet is very easy. It just takes a bit of preparation. If you do not know what Kale is, or where you would find Green Tea, then you may have a learning curve, albeit very small. There is little in the way of starting the Sirtfood diet.

Since you will be preparing and cooking healthy foods, you may want to do a few things the week you start:

1. Clear your cabinets and refrigerator of foods that are obviously unhealthy and that might tempt you. You also will have a very low calorie intake at the start, and you do not want to be tempted into a quick fix that may set you back. Even though you will have new recipes, you may feel that your old comfort foods are easier at the moment.

2. Go shopping for all of the ingredients that you will need for the week. If you buy what you will need it is more cost effective. Also, once you see the recipes, you will notice that there are many ingredients that overlap. You will get to know your portions as you proceed with the diet but at least you will have what you need and save yourself some trips to the store.

3. Wash, dry, cut and store all of the foods that you need, that way you have them conveniently prepared when you need them. This will make a new diet seem less tedious.

One necessary kitchen tool that you will need aside from the actual foods is a juicer. You will need a juicer as soon as you start the Sirtfood diet. Juicers are everywhere so they are quite easy to find, but the quality ranges greatly however. This is where price, function, and convenience comes into play. You could go to a popular department store, or you can find them online. Once you know what you are going after, you can shop around.

The quality of the juicer will also determine the nutritional quality and sometimes the taste of your juice. Just know that buying a cheap juicer may seem like a good idea now, but if you decide to upgrade later you will have spent more money, and twice. If you buy a good juicer, think of it like an investment into your health. Many people have spent money for a gym membership that went unused for quadruple the cost of one juicer. A juicer won't go to waste.

So, since not all juicers are alike, let us list a few of the features that you want to look for.

Centrifugal juicers:

Centrifugal juicers do just that, they use centrifugal force to spin the food (most like vegetables like carrots, cucumbers, or kale leaves) at high speeds to the side walls, where there are blades. The food is pushed through a sieve and then you have your juice. You have to drink this rather quickly, as you will lose nutrients the longer it is exposed to air (which it already has done as it was spinning), and it oxidizes, as well as a bit of heat from the friction which creates a loss of nutrients and enzymes. This is the whole reason you are juicing, so this point is quite important. You are also left with a lot of solid but very wet pulp as a byproduct, which also means there was a lot of fibrous parts of the plants that the juicer couldn't handle. This is also a missed opportunity for more nutrients. You will also get a lot of (warmish) foam at the top, which some people do not like. It is quick and it is easy however, and it is usually the cheapest of the juicer types. If you must it is better than not having one at all, but if you can make an investment, you will reap your rewards later.

Masticating juicers:

Masticating juicers also do what they say they are. They masticate or chew the food, albeit more slowly than the other type, by pulling it through gears which extract the juice. The machine pushes the pulp out. You would have less pulp with this machine afterwards. There is also less oxidation, and thus, more nutrients. They also can handle other types of foods (which varies by make and model), but that is something you should consider. You will get some foam with this as well, but not as much. These are more expensive, and again, should be looked at as you would an investment that you would not use and toss away. If you want it to last, and you want to get the most from your juicing and take it seriously, you will want to spend a bit more money and get what you really need.

Twin-gear/triturating juicers:

These geared juicers have gears that grind together with millimeters of space left between, to really tear open foods and grind the plants with only a very dry pulp that is left. These are the most nutrient-efficient juicers on the market. They leave virtually no foam and they are nutrient-dense as they are not disturbing the inner plant cells with oxidation. You usually can tell in the look (color) and taste (richer) than other juices. You can use different attachments to make different foods with most brands as well, so they are versatile. These are the highest pricing of most of the juicers in general, and there are also brand variations as with the others.

Citrus Juicers

There are also juicers specifically for citrus fruits. These can range from hand held, col-press juicers, to small electric or automatic cold-press juicers. They too vary in quality and price,

You can do a bit of research on the juicers that you may need. It will help engage your more in the process and journey you are about to take!

Storing Juices

The most nutrition from them immediately, you should drink them right away. If needed you can pre-juice, and put them in glass jelly, Mason jars. The wide mouth variety with the plastic lids is good, airtight and non-corrosive.

You can chill your drinks for the day, by resting them on ice packs in an insulated lunch tote or cooler. In extreme cases, you could juice one to three days of them (it is recommended at the maximum for optimal freshness, although you could push it further out

You may also find something to keep the juice chilled even while you are drinking at home. You can put a jar in the refrigerator just before prepping, and after you juice, pour it into one. You can make it a regular ritual of sorts. Have "your glass" that you get ready every day. If you prefer straws, you can even buy yourself a nice, reusable glass straw. None of these things are necessary for the diet, but any juice just tastes so much better when it is not from plastic.

Here are some other tips to help you get started:

Drink your juices as the earlier meals in the day if it helps you. It is a great way to start your day for three reasons.

- It will give you energy for breakfast and for lunch especially. By not having to digest heavy foods, your body saves time and energy usually spent on moving things around to go through all the laborious motions. You will be guaranteed to feel lighter and more energetic this way. You can always change this pattern after the maintenance phase, but you may find that you want to keep that schedule.

- Having fruits and vegetables before starchy or cooked meals, no matter how healthy the ingredients, is the best way to go for your digestion. Fruits and vegetables digest more rapidly, and the breakdown into the compounds that we can use more readily. Think of it as having your salad before your dinner. It works in the same way. The heavier foods, grains, oils, meats, etc., take more time to digest. If you eat these first, they will slow things down and that is where you have a backup of food needing to be broken down. This is also when you may find yourself with indigestion.

- Juices, especially green juices contain phytochemicals that not only serve as anti-oxidants but they contribute to our energy and mood. You will notice that you feel much differently after drinking a green juice than you would if you had eggs and sausage. You may want to make a food diary and note things such as this!

Be prepared to adjust to having lighter breakfasts for a little while. Most often we fill up with high protein, carbohydrate, and high calorie meals early in the day. We may feel that we did not get enough to eat and that we are not full at first. Oddly as it sounds, we may even miss the action of chewing. Some people need to chew their food to feel like they have had a filling meal. It is something automatic that we do not think of. Some also will miss that crunch such as with toast. Just pay attention to this, and know this is normal, and that it will pass.

Let's get started!

Chapter 1 Phase 1: The Slimming

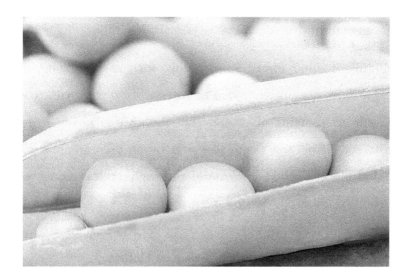

This is the period of hyper-success, where you are going to take a big step towards achieving a slimmer and leaner body. Follow our simple step-by-step instructions and use the delicious recipes you'll get. We do have a meat-free option in addition to our regular seven-day schedule, 0, which is ideal for vegetarians and vegans alike. Feel free to go along with whatever you want.

WHAT TO EXPECT

You will reap the full benefit of our clinically proven method of losing 7 pounds in seven days during Phase 1. But note that involves adding muscle, so don't just get caught up with the numbers on the. Nor should you become used to weighing yourself every day. In fact, in the last few days of Phase 1, we often see the scales creeping due to muscle gain, while waistlines continue to shrink. Therefore we want you to look at the scales but not be controlled by them. Find out how you look in the mirror, how you tingle your clothes, or if you need to push a knot on your belt. These are all perfect measures of the bigger changes in your body makeup.

Be mindful of other improvements, too, such as well-being, energy levels, and how smooth your skin is. At your local pharmacy, you can even get measurements of your overall cardiovascular and metabolic health to see changes in things like your blood pressure, blood sugar levels, and blood fats like cholesterol and triglycerides. Know, weight loss aside, incorporating Sirtfoods into your diet is a big step towards tightening your cells and making them more resistant to disease, setting you up for an exceptionally balanced lifetime.

How To Follow Phase 1

In order to make Phase 1 as smooth sailing as possible, we will direct you one day at a time through the complete seven-day plan, including the lowdown on the Sirtfood green juice and easy-to-follow, delicious recipes at every stage.

Phase 1 of the Sirtfood Diet is based on two distinct stages:

Days 1 to 3 are the most intensive, and during this time, you will consume up to a limit of 1,000 calories per day, consisting of:

- 3 x Sirtfood green juices
- 1 x main meal

Days 4 to 7 will see your daily consumption rise to a maximum of 1,500 calories, consisting of:

- 2 x Sirtfood green juices

- 2 x main meals

Ultimately, for sustained success, it's about tying it into the lifestyle and around daily life. But here are a few easy but big-impact tips to get the best result:

1. Get a Decent Juicer: Juicing is an important part of the Sirtfood Diet, and a juicer is one of the best investments you'll make for your wellbeing. Though the budget should be the deciding factor, some juicers are more efficient at extracting the juice from green leafy vegetables and herbs, with the Breville brand among the best juicers we've tried.

2. Preparation Is Key: One thing is evident from the abundance of feedback we've had: the most effective were those who prepared ahead of time. Get to know the ingredients and recipes and stock up on what's needed. You'll be surprised at how simple the whole process is, with everything planned and ready.

3. Save Time: Prepare cleverly when you're tight on time. Meals can be made the previous night. Juices can be made in bulk and stored in the refrigerator for up to three days (or longer in the freezer) until their sirtuin-activating nutrient levels begin to

fall. Just shield it from light, and add only when you're ready to eat it in the matcha.

4. Eat Early: Eating earlier in the day is safer, and preferably, meals and juices should not be eaten later than 7 p.m., but the diet is ideally built to suit your lifestyle, and late eaters often reap great bene t.

5. Stretch Out the Juices: They should be eaten at least one hour before or two hours after a meal to maximize the absorption of green juices and distributed throughout the day, rather than being too close together.

6. Eat until Satisfied: Sirtfoods can have drastic effects on appetite, and some people will be complete before they nest. Listen to your body and feed until you are full rather than forcing down all food. Tell "Hara Hachi bu," as the long-lived Okinawans do, which loosely translates as "Eat until you're 80 percent full."

7. Enjoy the Ride: Don't get stuck on the end goal, but remain conscious of the ride instead. This diet is about enjoying food in all its glory because of its health, but for the joy and enjoyment it brings. Research indicates that we are much more likely to succeed if we keep our minds focused on the road rather than the final goal.

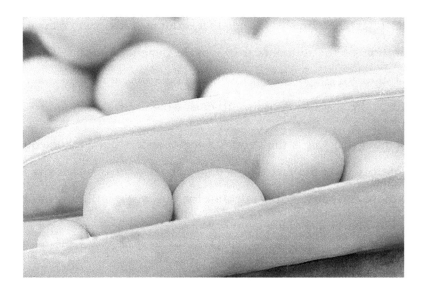

What To Drink

As well as the recommended daily portions of green juices, other fluids can be consumed free throughout Phase 1. Non-calorie beverages, preferably plain juice, black coffee, and green tea. If your usual tastes are for black or herbal teas, do not hesitate to include these too. Fruit juices and soft drinks are left behind. Instead, consider adding some sliced strawberries to still or sparkling water to make your own Sirtfood-infused health drink, if you want to spice things up. Hold it for a few hours in the fridge, and you will have a surprisingly soothing alternative to soft drinks and juices.

One thing you need to be aware of is that we don't suggest sudden major changes to your daily coffee use. Caffeine withdrawal symptoms may make you feel lousy for a few days; likewise, large increases may be unpleasant for those especially sensitive to caffeine effects. We also recommend that coffee be drunk black, without adding milk, because some researchers have found that adding milk can reduce the absorption of the nutrients that activate beneficial sirtuin. The same was found for green tea, although adding some lemon juice actually increases the absorption of its nutrients, which activate sirtuin.

Remember that this is the period of hyper-success, and while you can be comforted by the fact that it is just for a week, you need to be a little more careful. We have alcohol for this week, in the form of red wine but only as a cooking ingredient.

THE SIRTFOOD GREEN JUICE

Green juice is an integral part of Sirtfoods phase 1 diet. All the ingredients are strong Sirtfoods, and in every juice, you get a potent cocktail of natural compounds like apigenin, kaempferol, luteolin, quercetin, and EGCG that work together to turn on your sirtuin genes and promote fat loss. To that, we have added lemon, as it has been shown that its natural acidity prevents, stabilizes, and increases the absorption of the sirtuin-activating nutrients. We added a bit of apple and ginger to taste too. But both of these are optional. Indeed, a lot of people and that once they're used to juice flavor, they leave the apple out altogether.

Chapter 2 Phase 2: - The Maintenance

Congrats on completing Phase 1 of the Sirtfood Diet! As of now, you must be seeing top-notch results with fats misfortune and are not handiest looking slimmer and progressively conditioned, anyway feeling revived and reenergized. All in all, what now?

Having seen those regularly significant alterations ourselves firsthand, we understand the amount you'll have to not merely hold all the one's benefits, anyway, observe stunningly better results. Sirtfoods are intended to be eaten forever. The inquiry is how you adjust what you have been doing in Phase 1 into your common dietary repeating. That is what initiated us to make a subsequent fourteen-day remodel plan intended to assist you with making the change from Phase 1 to your additional ordinary dietary daily practice and therefore help keep up and also increment the benefits of the Sirtfood Diet.

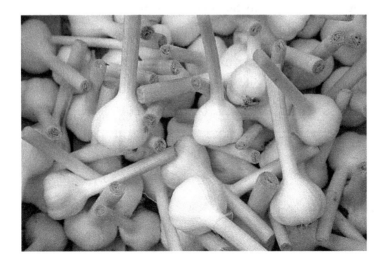

What's in store?

During Phase 2, you will merge your weight reduction outcomes and hold them to get in shape consistently.

Recollect that the central striking angle we have found with the Sirtfood Diet is that greatest or the entirety of the weight that individuals lose is from fats, and that numerous genuinely put on a couple of muscle. So we have to remind you again now not to pick your advancement absolutely by methods for the numbers on the scale.

Recall too that primarily as the weight reduction will save, the wellness benefits will develop. By following the fourteen-day protection plan, you're entirely beginning to put down the standards for a fate of profoundly rooted wellbeing.

The most effective method to FOLLOW PHASE 2

The way to accomplishment in this stage is to keep up pressing you're eating routine loaded with Sirtfoods. To make it as spotless as could reasonably be expected, we've assembled a seven-day menu plan which will follow, including flavorful family-accommodating projects, with consistently pressed to the rafters with Sirtfoods (however observe page 149 for guidance concerning kids). You should simply rehash the seven-day procedure twice to complete the fourteen days of Phase 2.

On every one of the fourteen days your weight-reduction plan will comprise of:

- Three x adjusted Sirtfood-rich suppers

- 1 x Sirtfood green juice

- 1 to 2 x non-mandatory Sirtfood piece snacks

Indeed, there are no unbending guidelines for on the off chance that you need to eat up these. Be flexible and t them around your day. Two simple instructions of thumb are:

Have your green juice both first viewpoint in the first part of the day, as a base thirty minutes before breakfast, or midmorning.

Try your phenomenal to eat up your night supper employing 7 p.m.

Part SIZES

Our concentration for the length of Phase 2 isn't generally on checking calories. Over the drawn-out, this isn't always a viable or perhaps fruitful methodology for the regular individual. Instead, we're concentrating on reasonable bits, much adjusted food, and most extreme significance, filling up on Sirtfoods so you can keep on benefit from their fats-consuming and wellness selling results.

We have furthermore constructed the dinners inside the arrangement to make them satisfying, to have the option to assist you with encountering full for more. That,

mixed with the grown home hunger controlling aftereffects of Sirtfoods, implies which you won't go through the following fourteen days feeling hungry, anyway as an option enjoyably satisfied, appropriately took care of, and phenomenally appropriately sustained.

Similarly, as in Phase 1, remember to tune in to your body and be guided by your craving. If you get ready food with regards to our orders and you're serenely finished sooner than you've finished dinner, at that point, it's impeccably done to quit ingesting!

WHAT TO DRINK

You will hold to envelop one unpracticed squeeze step by step throughout Phase 2. This is to keep you bested up with over the top levels of Sirtfoods.

Similarly, as in Phase 1, you could eat diverse guides openly all through Phase 2. Our favored beverages while in transit to comprise of keep on being plain water, independent favored water, espresso, and green tea. On the off chance that your preference is for dark or white tea, experience free to delight in. The equivalent applies to healthy drinks. The top-notch data is that you may appreciate the occasional glass of red wine during Phase 2. Red wine is a Sirtfood because of its substance material of sirtuin-initiating polyphenols, specifically resveratrol and piceatannol, making it by methods for far the best want of mixed refreshment. Yet, with liquor itself having conflicting results on our fats cells, balance is still high-caliber. Throughout Phase 2, we prescribe confining your admission to 1 glass of ruby wine with a dinner, on or three days as indicated by week.

Coming back TO THREE MEALS

During Phase 1, you expended essentially one or dinners daily, which gave you masses of flexibility over while you ate your suppers. As we presently come back to a more prominent regular customary and the time-demonstrated example of 3 suppers per day, it's a decent time to discuss breakfast.

We have an astonishing breakfast unit us up for the afternoon, developing our power and mindfulness stages. Regarding our digestion, eating ahead of time proceeds with our glucose and fats levels under tight restraints. That breakfast is an essential component is borne out by utilizing various examinations that ordinarily show that people that habitually eat up breakfast are considerably less liable to be overweight.

The reason for this is because of our inward casing timekeepers (see page 72). Our bodies anticipate that we should eat right off the bat, fully expecting when we will be generally dynamic and needing fuel. However, on some random day, upwards of a third person will skip breakfast. It's a common side effect of our bustling contemporary lives, and the conviction is that there sincerely isn't sufficient opportunity to devour well. In any case, as you'll see, with the quick morning meals we have spread out for you here, nothing might need to be further from reality. Regardless of whether it's the Sirtfood smoothie that can be affected by liquor in a hurry, the premade Sirt muesli, or the short and clean Sirtfood fried eggs/tofu, finding the ones more prominent couple of moments inside the morning will get profits not, at this point best in your day yet to your more extended term weight and wellbeing.

With Sirtfoods working to supercharge our vitality levels, there might be significantly more noteworthy to be gotten from getting an early morning hit of them to begin your day. This is accomplished not through merely expending a Sirtfood-well off breakfast, anyway primarily through the consideration of the green juice, which we embrace you have both the first segment inside the morning—as a base thirty minutes before breakfast—or midmorning. From our own clinical experience, we do get numerous surveys of individuals who drink their green juice component and don't feel hungry for over one hour a short time later. On the off chance that this is the effect it has on you, it is superbly done to hold up two or three hours sooner than eating. Simply don't pass it. On the other hand, you may commence your day with a decent breakfast, at that point, pause or 3 hours before having the green juice. Be flexible and go together with something that works for you.

SIRT FOOD BITES

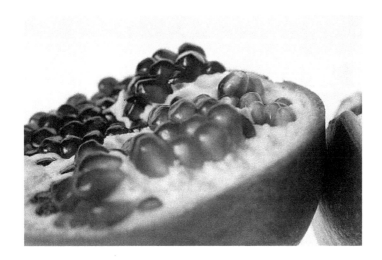

Concerning nibbling, you could accept the only choice available. There has been a great deal banter about in the case of eating regular, littler dinners are decent for weight reduction, or whether you should simply adhere to 3 adjusted suppers daily. In all actuality, it doesn't genuinely make a difference.

The way we have developed the remodel menu for you guarantees you will devour three even Sirtfood-rich dinners in sync with day, as a general rule don't need a bite. In any case, potentially you've been occupied in the office, running out, or running around with the children, and need something to hold you over to the accompanying supper. Furthermore, if that "small something" is going to give you a whammy of Sirtfood nutrients and taste scrumptious, at that point, its glad days. It is the reason we made our "Sirtfood nibbles."

Chapter 3 Phase 1 Diet (Day 1-4)

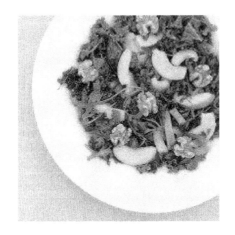

DAY 1

BREAKFAST

(ALSO SUITABLE FOR MID-MORNING SNACK OR AFTERNOON TEA)

Green Juice

Preparation time: 10 minutes

Cooking time: 0 minutes

Servings: 2

Ingredients:

75g Kale

30 g arugula

10 g parsley

150 g celery

Medium green apple

Lemon

½ teaspoon matcha green tea

Tablespoon agave or natural honey (optional)

Directions:

Clean the vegetables and fruit. Put the kale, arugula and parsley in the juicier or blender. Add some water if you are using a blender.

Next, Juice the celery and apple.

Squeeze the lemon into the resulting juice above.

Use a fine mesh strainer to strain the juice it you like. This is optional.

Pour some juice into a glass and add the matcha green tea. Stir to dissolve completely. Then top up with the rest of the juice. If using a blender, add the green tea into the blender and blitz foe a few second.

You may add some water to the green juice before drinking.

Nutrition:

Calories: 18 Net carbs: 20.6g Fat: 0.5g Fiber: 4.2g Protein: 1.8g

LUNCH

Chicken Stir-Fry (1 Serving)

Preparation time: 10 minutes

Cooking time: 30 minutes

Servings: 1

Ingredients:

1 boneless and skinless chicken breast (about 120 g, sliced thinly)

50 g buckwheat or buckwheat noodle (soba)

100 g kale (cleaned and chopped)

1 small red onion (peeled and chopped)

1 clove garlic (peeled and chopped)

½ inch ginger root (peeled and sliced) 1 teaspoon turmeric

Some parsley (as a garnish)

1 or more bird's eye chili (optional) ½ lemon (optional)

1-2 tablespoon extra-virgin olive oil Seasonings: salt, pepper, sesame oil, soy sauce or tamari sauce, oyster Sauce, etc.

Directions:

Marinate the chicken with the turmeric powder and some salt. Pepper and soy sauce. Just add a bit of the seasonings as you will adjust the taste again later.

Cook the buckwheat/ buckwheat noodle according to the packet instructions.

Heat a large work or frying pan. Add the kale with some sale water. Cook it for a few minutes until it wilts. Take it out and cool under running water to keep the color.

Dry the wok or pan and heat up the olive oil. Add the red onion, garlic and ginger. Stir fry for a few minutes.

Add the chicken and the chili into the wok. Cook them until brown or done.

Add some water to create some sauce or gravy (add more to get a nice gravy). Bring the mixture to a simmer. Adjust the taste again by adding some seasonings like soy sauce, sesame oil, oyster sauce, etc.

Add in the kale. If you are using buckwheat noodle, you can also add the noodles to the chicken mixture. Coat everything with thee sauce.

Take out and garnish with the chopped parsley. Squeeze the lemon if using.

Nutrition:

Calories: 186

Net carbs: 4.6 g

Fat: 2.9 g

DINNER

Green Juice. Use the same recipe as above.

DAY 2

BREAKFAST

(ALSO SUITABLE FOR MID-MORNING SNACK OR AFTERNOON TEA)

Berry Juice

Preparation time: 10 minutes

Cooking time: 0 minutes

Servings: 1-2

Ingredients:

1 cup strawberries

1 cup blueberries

1 green apple (cored and cut)

50 g celery

1-2 stalks parsley

½ lemon

½ teaspoon matcha green tea

Directions:

Clean the vegetables and fruit. Juice or blend the fruits and vegetables.

Squeeze the lemon into the resulting juice above.

Use a fine mesh strainer to strain the juice if you like. This is optional.

Pour some juice into a glass and add the matcha green tea. Stir to dissolve completely. Then top up with the rest of the juice. If using a blender, add the green tea into the blender and blitz for a few seconds.

You may add some water to dilute the juice before drinking.

Nutrition:

Calories: 74

Net carbs: 6.4g

Fat: 10g

Fiber: 1.3g

Protein: 17.3g

LUNCH

Tuna Salad

Preparation time: 5 minutes

Cooking time: 0 minutes

Servings: 1

Ingredients: ½ of a can of tuna (tuna in brine/water or oil)

1 small red onion (peeled and chopped) Salt& pepper

50 g arugula/rocket (more or less to your liking)

50 g red chicory (more or less to your liking)

2 medjool dates (pitted and chopped) 30 g celery (chopped or sliced

1-2 stalks parsley (chopped) 1 tablespoon capers

1 tablespoon extra-virgin olive oil 1 tablespoon lemon juice

Directions:

Drain and flake the tuna. Clean and chopped the vegetables.

Mix all the ingredients in a large salad bowl. Enjoy.

Nutrition:

Calories: 383 Net carbs: 14.4g Fat: 22.9g Fiber: 0.8g Protein: 29.6g

DINNER

Berry Juice. Use the same recipe as above.

DAY 3

BREAKFAST

Green Juice With Blueberries

(ALSO SUITABLE FOR MID-MORNING SNACK OR AFTERNOON TEA)

Preparation time: 10 minutes

Cooking time: 0 minutes

Servings: 1-2

Ingredients:

1 cup blueberries 1 green apple (cored and cut)

50 g celery 75 g kale Cucumber (peeled and cut)

Directions:

Clean the vegetables and fruits. Juice or blend the fruits and vegetables.

Use a fine mesh strainer to strain the juice if you like. This is optional.

You may add some water to dilute the juice before drinking.

Nutrition:

Calories: 85 Net carbs: 29.7g Fat: 0.8g

Fiber: 5.2g Protein: 3.2g

LUNCH

Tofu-Veggie Stir-Fry

Preparation time: 5 minutes

Cooking time: 10 minutes

Servings: 1-2

Ingredients:

14-0unce package firm or extra-firm tofu (can replace tofu with lean Chicken/turkey) 1 cup kale 1 cup rocket or arugula

1 small red onion (peeled and chopped) 1 clove garlic (minced)

A small handful walnuts (chopped) Stalk parsley (chopped)

1 tablespoon extra-virgin olive oil 1-2 bird's eye chili (optional)

50 g buckwheat or buckwheat noodle (prepared according to the packet instructions

Seasoning5: salt, pepper, sesame oil, soy sauce or tamari sauce, oyster sauce, chili sauce, etc.

Directions:

Pre-heat the oven to 400 "F.

Take half of the tofu and place between two clean towels or several layers of paper towels to dry the tofu.

When it is dry, roughly cut it into 1inch cubes.

Arrange the tofu on parchment-lined baking sheet and bake for 25- 35 minutes. Flip them once halfway through the baking. Baking the tofu will dry it up and produce a moat-like texture. If you prefer an even firmer texture, continue baking for another 10 minutes or more. Just don't burn the tofu. If you are using lean chicken or turkey instead of tofu, skip step 1-4. Stir fry the chicken in the wok or pan.

Heat a large wok or frying pan. Add the kale with some water. Cook it for a few minutes until it wilts. Take it out and cool under running water to keep the color.

Dry the pan and heat up the oil in the pan. Add the garlic and onion. Fry them for about 2 minutes.

Add the tofu into the pan. Add some water, about 1/3 cup to produce some gravy. Add your preferred seasonings such as soy sauce, oyster sauce and chili sauce

Add in the kale and arugula. Simmer for about 1 - 2 minutes.

Dish out and garnish with the chopped walnuts and parsley.

Serve with the prepared buckwheat.

Nutrition:

Calories: 186 Net carbs: 33g Fat: 16.9g Fiber: 1.2g Protein: 6.4g

DINNER

Green Juice with Blueberries. Follow the recipe above.

DAY 4

BREAKFAST

Kale Smoothie

(ALSO SUITABLE FOR MID-MORNING SNACK OR AFTERNOON TEA)

Preparation time: 10 minutes

Cooking time: 0 minutes

Servings: 1

Ingredients:

50g kale or 1 cup packed 30g celery Green apple 1 handful blueberries

½ cucumber (peeled and cut) ½ teaspoon matcha green tea

Directions:

Juice or blend all the ingredients except the green tea. Add the green tea at the end and blitz for a few seconds.

Use a fine mesh strainer to strain the juice before drinking (optional). Top-up with water if needed.

Nutrition:

Calories: 186 Net carbs: 7.8g Fat: 7.8g Fiber: 8.5g Protein: 10.7g

LUNCH

Teriyaki Salmon

Preparation time: 10 minutes

Cooking time: 0 minutes

Servings: 2

Ingredients:

2 salmon filets (medium size)

1 clove garlic (minced

1/8 teaspoon grated ginger root

2 small red onions (chopped)

2 tablespoons light soy sauce

1 ½ tablespoon maple syrup/agave/natural honey

1 tablespoon mixing /rice wine

1 ½ tablespoons extra-virgin olive oil

2 stalks chopped parsley (for garnishing)

Salt and pepper

Directions:

Prepare the dressing by mixing the garlic, grated ginger, onion, soy sauce, maple syrup, mixing and halt tablespoon olive oil in a bowl.

Season the salmon fillets with salt and pepper. Pour the prepared dressing over the salmons and coat evenly: Cover and keep in the refrigerator to marinate for at least 1 hour,

Heat one tablespoon of the olive oil in a non-stick pan. Add the salmon, skin side down and cook for about 2 minutes.

Pour the marinade over the salmon. Add some water to the pan and baste the salmons with the sauce. Cook for about 2 minutes until the salmons turn opaque halfway up the sides.

Turn the salmons over to cook the other side for 3 4 minutes. Keep basting with the sauce. Add more water if the sauce is too thick. Adjust the seasoning if necessary.

Dish out the salmons. Garnish with the chopped parsley. Enjoy 1 fillet far lunch and reserve the other for dinner.

Serve the salmon with cooked buckwheat or an Apple Walnut Salad.

Nutrition:

Calories: 186

Net carbs: 13.8g

Fat: 13.7g

Fiber: 0.3g

Protein: 40.9g

LUNCH

Apple Walnut Salad

Preparation time: 10 minutes

Cooking time: 0 minutes

Servings: 1-2

Ingredients: 1 green apple (cored and diced/sliced)

1 small red onion (diced) 50 g celery (diced or sliced thinly)

50 g rocket/arugula (or 1 cup packed) 1 tomato (diced or sliced)

¼ cup walnuts (chopped) ½ cup medjool dates (pitted and chopped)

1 teaspoon maple syrup/agave/natural honey

1 tablespoon lemon juice

1 tablespoons reduced-calorie mayonnaise/non-fat sour cream

1 stalk chopped parsley (for garnishing) Salt and pepper

Directions:

Mix the apples with the lemon juice in a bowl. Add the celery, walnuts, tomato, onion, dates and rocket. Mix the mayonnaise with the syrup and fold into the salad mixture. Season with salt and pepper. Garnish with the chopped parsley.

Nutrition: Calories: 186   Net carbs: 10.5g Fat: 10.4g Fiber: 2.3g Protein: 1.5g

DINNER

Enjoy the second portion of the salmon. Serve with Apple Walnut Salad, cooked buckwheat or other simple salad.

Chapter 4 Phase 1 Diet (Day 5-7)

DAY 5

BREAKFAST

Pita

Preparation time: 5 minutes

Cooking time: 10 minutes

Servings: 1

Ingredients:

1 pita whole-meal pita bread (6 inch-diameter)

1 tomato (diced)

1 small red onion (chopped)

50 g rocket/arugula or 1 cup packed

1 stalk parsley/lavage (chopped)

1 tablespoon capers

1 tablespoon grated parmesan cheese

¼ cup feta cheese/shredded mozzarella cheese

Salt and pepper

Directions:

Heat ne oven to broil and arrange a rack in the middle.

Place the pita on a broiler pan and sprinkle with the feta/mozzarella cheese. Arrange the rocket over the cheese. Leave a small space in the center of the pita.

Crack an egg into the center of the pita. Sprinkle over with the red onion, tomato, caper, olive oil, salt and pepper.

Broil the pita until the egg white has set, about 6- 7 minutes (your preference).

Remove the pan iron the oven and transfer the pita to a plate. Sprinkle with the parmesan cheese and garnish with the parsley/lavage.

Nutrition:

Calories: 186

Net carbs: 25g

Fat: 0.5g

Fiber: 1g

Protein: 4.1g

LUNCH

Refreshing Green Juice

(ALSO SUITABLE FOR MID-MORNING SNACK OR AFTERNOON TEA)

Preparation time: 10 minutes

Cooking time: 0 minutes

Servings: 1-2

Ingredients:

50g kale or rocket (or 1 cup packed) 1 green apple (cut and cared)

150g celery ½ lemon ½ teaspoon matcha green tea

½ cucumber (peeled and cut)

Directions:

Blend or blitz all the ingredients except the lemon and green tea. Squeeze the lemon into the mixture and add the green tea. Blitz for a few seconds.

Use a fine mesh strainer to strain the juice before drinking (optional). Top up with water if desired.

Nutrition:

Calories: 186 Net carbs: 14.1g Fat: 0.6g Fiber: 1.4g Protein:1.7g

DINNER

Meat Loaf Pita Sandwich

Preparation time: 10 minutes

Cooking time: 0 minutes

Servings: 1

Ingredients:

1 meat loaf 1 whole meal pita bread (6 inch-diameter)

1 tomato (diced) 1 small red onion (chopped)

1 stalk parsley/lavage (chopped) 50 g rocket/arugula (or 1 cup packed)

1 tablespoon lemon juice 1 tablespoon extra-virgin olive oil

¼ crumbled feta cheese (optional) Salt and pepper

Directions:

Reheat the meat loaf in the microwave. Slice or crumble the meat loaf and divide into two portions

Mix the tomato, onion, parsley/lavage, rocket, olive oil, lemon juice, salt and pepper. Stir In the feta cheese.

Cut the pita bread in half. Stuff each half with a mixture of meat loaf and the salad above. Enjoy.

Nutrition:

Calories: 186 Net carbs: 1.2g Fat: 4.1g Protein: 4.1g

DAY 6

BREAKFAST

Soy Berry Smoothie

(ALSO SUITABLE FOR MID-MORNING SNACK OR AFTERNOON TEA)

Preparation time: 10 minutes

Cooking time: 0 minutes

Servings: 1

Ingredients:

1 cup fresh strawberries/blueberries (or frozen)

1 cup unsweetened vanilla soymilk

Directions:

Blend or blitz all the ingredients. Enjoy.

Nutrition:

Calories: 186

Net carbs: 112g

Fat: 3.4g

Fiber:32.9g

Protein: 18.9g

OR

Berry Yoghurt

Preparation time: 5 minutes

Cooking time: 0 minutes

Servings: 1

Ingredients:

½ cup vanilla fat-free yoghurt

½ cup strawberries/blueberries

Directions:

Mix all the ingredients. Enjoy.

Nutrition:

Calories: 186

Net carbs: 22.5g

Fat: 1.2g

Fiber: 1.1g

Protein: 3g

LUNCH

Lentil Curry

Preparation time: 24 hours

Cooking time: 30 minutes

Servings: 1

Ingredients:

50g rod or yellow lentils

1 large potato or sweet potato (peeled and cubed)

1 clove garlic (minced)

1 medium red onion or 3 small red onions (chopped) tomato (quartered) tablespoons turmeric

1 tablespoon curry paste/powder

2 cups vegetable/chicken broth

½ cup low fat milk

½ cup plain yoghurt (non-fat)

1 teaspoon cooking oil

2 stalks parsley (for garnishing)

Salt and pepper

Directions:

Prepare the lentils the day before (on Day 2). Place the lentils in a sieve or colander and rinse under running tap water. Put the lentils inside a bowl/container and add enough tap water to cover the top. Cover the bowl/container and refrigerate. Leave it to soak overnight. This will soften and shorten the cooking time. It is not a problem if you skip this stop. The cooking time will be slightly longer.

Heat the oil in a pot and add the garlic and onion. Fry for about 2-3 minutes.

Drain the lentils and add it to the pot. Add the tomato, potato, turmeric and curry spices. Fry for about 2 minutes.

Pour in the vegetable broth and milk. Add same seasonings

Bring the mixture to a boil, then reduce to a simmer. Simmer the mixture for 20-30 minutes or until the lentils and potato0s have soften.

Add more liquid if you want it more 'soupy.' Also add the yoghurt. Add more seasonings if necessary.

Divide the curry into 2 portions. Enjoy one portion for lunch and the next for dinner

Serve the curry with cooked buckwheat if you like.

Nutrition:

Calories: 186 Net carbs: 10.4g Fat: 1g Fiber: 2.3g Protein: 4g

DINNER

Lentil Curry

Enjoy the second portion of the lentil curry. Serve with cooked buckwheat or a salad.

Day 7

BREAKFAST

Matcha Apple & Green Juice

Preparation Time: 10 minutes

Cooking time: 0 minutes

Servings: 2

Ingredients:

5 ounces fresh kale

2 ounces fresh arugula

¼ cup fresh parsley

4 celery stalks

1 green apple, cored and chopped

1 (1-inch) piece fresh ginger, peeled

1 lemon, peeled

½ teaspoon matcha green tea

Directions:

Add all ingredients into a juicer and extract the juice according to the manufacturer's method.

Pour into two glasses and serve immediately.

Nutrition:

Calories: 113

Net carbs: 31.7g

Fat: 0.2g

Fiber: 0.2g

Protein: 0.6g

LUNCH

Chickpeas With Swiss Chard

Preparation Time: 15 minutes

Cooking Time: 12 minutes

Servings: 4

Ingredients:

2 tablespoon olive oil

2 garlic cloves, sliced thinly

1 large tomato, chopped finely

2 bunches fresh Swiss chard, trimmed

1 (18-ounce) can chickpeas, drained and rinsed

Salt and ground black pepper, as required

¼ cup water

1 tablespoon fresh lemon juice

2 tablespoons fresh parsley, chopped

Directions:

Heat the oil in a large nonstick wok over medium heat and sauté the garlic for about 1 minute.

Add the tomato and cook for about 2-3 minutes, crushing with the back of spoon.

Stir in remaining ingredients except lemon juice and parsley and cook for about 5-7 minutes.

Drizzle with the lemon juice and remove from the heat.

Serve hot with the garnishing of parsley.

Nutrition:

Calories: 217 Net carbs: 8.6g Fat: 1.3g Fiber: 4.5g Protein: 4.3g

DINNER

Shrimp With Veggies

Preparation Time: 15 minutes

Cooking Time: 8 minutes

Servings: 5

Ingredients:

For Sauce:

1 tablespoon fresh ginger, grated

2 garlic cloves, minced

3 tablespoons low-sodium soy sauce

1 tablespoon red wine vinegar

1 teaspoon brown sugar

¼ teaspoon red pepper flakes, crushed

For Shrimp Mixture:

3 tablespoons olive oil

1½ pounds medium shrimp, peeled and deveined

12 ounces broccoli florets

8 ounces, carrot, peeled and sliced

Directions:

For sauce: in a bow, place all the ingredients and beat until well combined. Set aside.

In a large wok, heat oil over medium-high heat and cook the shrimp for about 2 minutes, stirring occasionally.

Add the broccoli and carrot and cook about 3-4 minutes, stirring frequently.

Stir in the sauce mixture and cook for about 1-2 minutes.

Serve immediately.

Nutrition:

Calories 298

Net carbs: 1.5g

Fat: 1.6g

Fiber: 0.6g

Protein: 9.8g

Chapter 5 Phase Two Diet (First Three Days Of The Week)

DAY 8 and 15

BREAKFAST

Baked Eggs Over Avocado With Goat Cheese Or Bacon

Preparation time: 10 minutes

Cooking time: 15 minutes

Servings: 4

Ingredients:

2 Egg

2 Serrano ham slices

50g Onion

50g Mozzarella Cheese

Fresh parsley

Salt

Ground black pepper

Muffin or cupcake molds

Directions:

Grease each mold with butter and roll up a slice of Serrano ham in each one.

Chop the onion, a couple of branches of parsley and the mozzarella cheese.

Beat the eggs in a container and add the onion, parsley and cheese. Salt and pepper to taste.

Fill each mold with this mixture in such a way that it reaches the top of the mold and completely fills it.

Place the molds in the hot oven at 180°C for about 20 minutes. Once ready, remove from the oven and serve.

Nutrition:

Calories: 290

Net carbs: 12.9g

Fat: 31.5g

Fiber: 9.3g

Protein: 15.2g

LUNCH

Parmesan Chicory Zuppa

Preparation time: 10 minutes

Cooking time: 35 minutes

Servings: 4

Ingredients:

An Onion (chopped)

60g of celery (in fine cubes)

200g of parsnip (sliced)

1 Tablespoons of olive oil

2 Tablespoons spice mixture

1 Teaspoon rosemary

250g chicory, in strips)

100g of chickpeas (can)

1 Tablespoon mustard (spicy)

3rd Tablespoons milk

5 Tablespoons parmesan (freshly grated)

2nd Organic egg yolks

0.5 Juice oranges

Pepper (freshly ground)

Directions:

Braise the onion, celery and parsnips in olive oil. Add the spice mixture, rosemary and chicory (take a few vegetable strips for later) and add 600–800 ml of boiling water and cook over a medium heat for 8 minutes. Add drained chickpeas and heat in the soup for 5 minutes.

Mix the mustard, milk, 3 tablespoons of Parmesan cheese and egg yolk and alloy (bind) the soup with the mixture. Do not let the soup boil anymore and season with a few splashes of orange juice and pepper.

Arrange the soup and sprinkle with chicory and 1 tablespoon of Parmesan cheese.

Nutrition:

Calories: 385

Net carbs: 3g

Fat: 0.3g

Protein: 3g

DINNER

Turkey Kebab With Chakalaka

Preparation time: 10 minutes

Cooking time: 35 minutes

Servings: 4

Ingredients:

100g of organic turkey breast fillet

3rd teaspoon olive oil 1 TL (BBQ Rub spice mix)

80g papaya (in large pieces)

1 Onion (finely chopped)

1 Clove of garlic (finely chopped) 1 Tsp curry powder (mild)

1 Teaspoon ginger (frozen) 1 TL chili (TK)

200g of carrot (grated) 0.5 green peppers (diced)

1 Tsp agave syrup 0.5 Tsp cumin Salt

2nd Teaspoon tomato paste

150g of tomatoes (in cubes)

100g of legumes (frozen mixture, e.g. Mexican)

1 EL papaya (kernels)

2nd Tablespoons plain yogurt (3.8% fat)

Directions:

Preheat the oven to 180 degrees, convection 160 degrees, and gas level 3.

Dice the meat and mix with 1 teaspoon of olive oil and BBQ rub. Put the meat and papaya on wooden skewers and place on a baking sheet lined with baking paper.

For the chakalaka, braise the onion, garlic, curry, ginger and chili in 2 teaspoons of olive oil. Add carrots and peppers and stir-fry for 2-3 minutes. Season with agave syrup, cumin and salt. Add the tomato paste, tomatoes and frozen legumes and cook over a medium heat for 10–12 minutes.

Meanwhile, fry the skewers in the oven on the middle rail for 5 minutes on each side. Arrange with half of the chakalaka, garnish with yoghurt and papaya seeds. The rest of the chakalaka should be eaten the next day with fish, omelet or whole grain rice.

Nutrition:

Calories: 465

Fat: 15.6g

Protein:129g

Day 9 and 16

BREAKFAST

Berry Oat Breakfast Cobbler

Preparation time: 5 minutes

Cooking time: 45 minutes

Servings: 2

Ingredients:

2 cups of oats/flakes that are ready without cooking

1 cup of blackcurrants without the stems

1 teaspoon of honey (or ¼ teaspoon of raw sugar)

½ cup of water (add more or less by testing the pan)

1 cup of plain yogurt (or soy or coconut)

Directions:

Boil the berries, honey and water and then turn it down on low. Put in a glass container in a refrigerator until it is cool and set (about 30 minutes or more)

Nutrition:

Calories: 241 Net carbs: 42.7g Fat: 11.4g Fiber: 32.9g Protein: 18.9g

LUNCH

Baked Salmon Salad With Creamy Mint Dressing

Preparation time: 5 minutes

Cooking time: 10 minutes

Servings: 1

Ingredients:

1 fillet of salmon (130 g)

40g mixed leaves of salad

40g green leaves of spinach

2 radishes, cut and sliced thinly

5cm (50g) cucumber slice, split into bits

2 onions of spring, trimmed and sliced

1 tiny handful (10g) parsley, chopped roughly

For the Dressing

Low-fat mayonnaise 1 teaspoon

1 tablespoon of yogurt.

1 tablespoon vinegar of rice

2 mint leaves, finely cut.

Salt and black pepper freshly ground

Directions:

Preheat the oven to 180 ° C (200 ° C).

Put the fillet on a baking tray and bake it 16–18 minutes before the fillet has just been cooked. Take off the oven and set aside. The salmon in the salad is equally nice hot, or cold. If the salmon is skinny, just cook the meat and separate it from the meat with a fish slice. When cooked, it should slide off easily.

Combine the mayonnaise, yogurt, vinegar rice, mint leaves, and salt and pepper in a small bowl and let at least 5 minutes stand to enable the mixture to start.

Place the spinach and the salad leaves and the radishes, the cucumber, the spring onions and the parsley on the serving plate. Drop the salmon on the salad and drizzle on the sauce.

Nutrition:

Calories: 340

Net carbs: 0.4g

Fat: 1.2g

Protein: 22g

DINNER

Kale, Edamame And Tofu Curry

Preparation time: 10 minutes

Cooking time: 25 minutes

Servings: 2

Ingredients:

1 tablespoon rapeseed oil

One large onion, chopped

Four cloves garlic, peeled and grated

One large thumb (7cm) fresh ginger, peeled and grated

*One red chili, deseeded and thinly sliced

1/2 teaspoon ground turmeric

1/4 teaspoon cayenne pepper

1 teaspoon paprika

1/2 teaspoon ground cumin

1 teaspoon salt

250g dried red lentils

1 liter boiling water

50g frozen soya beans

200g firm tofu, chopped into cubes Two tomatoes, roughly chopped Juice of 1 lime 200g kale leaves stalk removed and torn

Directions:

Put the oil over low-medium heat in a heavy-bottomed oven. Add the onion and cook for 5 minutes before inserting the garlic, ginger, and chili, then simmer for another 2 minutes. Add the turmeric, cayenne, cumin, paprika, and salt. Remove and mix again, before introducing the red lentils.

Pour in the boiling water and cook for 10 minutes until the curry has a thick 'porridge' consistency, then reduce the heat and cook for another 20-30 minutes.

Remove the soya beans, tofu, and tomatoes and continue cooking for another 5 minutes. Add the juice of lime and kale leaves, then simmer until the kale is soft.

Place the buckwheat in a medium saucepan around 15 minutes until the curry is ready, and add plenty of boiling water. Bring the water back to the boil and cook for 10 minutes (or somewhat longer if you want softer buckwheat. Drain the buckwheat in a sieve and serve with the dhal.

Nutrition:

Calories: 342 Net carbs: 8.4g Fat: 17g Protein: 12.6g

Day 10 and 17

BREAKFAST

Mushroom Buckwheat Pancakes

Preparation time: 10 minutes

Cooking time: 30 minutes

Servings: 3

Ingredients:

55g whole meal flour

55g buckwheat flour

275ml Alpo Almond Milk

1 free-range egg

30g butter, for frying

For the Filling

50g flour

50g butter

275ml Alpo Almond Milk

1 free-range egg

100g sliced chestnut mushrooms

3 large handfuls of baby spinach

Olive oil 275ml Alpo Almond Milk 1 free-range egg

Directions:

Melt butter in a saucepan 50 g. Use the flour to create a paste. Continue cooking for 30 seconds.

Gradually add the milk, stirring vigorously until the white sauce is smooth. (Make sure to stir well so that lumps do not form.)

Fry the mushrooms in the oil until the spinach is brown and wilt. Drop the mushrooms into the white sauce, add the cheese and nutmeg to taste, then season.

In the meantime, add the two flour types to a bowl, and make a small well.

Whisk the egg into the milk, lightly. Pour a handful of the egg mixture into the flour and continue whisking. Start applying the liquid and whisking until the batter is smooth.

Melt the butter and add a ladle of the batter in a non-stick frying pan. Swirl to brush the base of the pan equally, then turn it as the pancake is shakable. Repeat until all the batter has been consumed, and then line it with mushroom and spinach stuffing.

Nutrition:

Calories: 337 Net carbs: 40 g Fat: 9.82g

Fiber: 6.2 g Protein: 32g

LUNCH

Asian King Prawn Stir-Fry With Buckwheat Noodles

Preparation time: 5 minutes

Cooking time: 20 minutes

Servings: 2

Ingredients:

150g of raw king creeping shell, deveined

2 teaspoon tamari (you can also use soy sauce)

Extra virgin olive oil 2 teaspoon additional

75g soba (noodles of buckwheat)

1 clove of garlic, finely minced

1 chili bird's head, thinly cut

1 teaspoon of new ginger finely minced

Sliced 20 g red onions

40g of celery, cut and sliced

75g of green beans, cut

Chicken reserve 100ml

50g spinach, sliced roughly

Celery leaves 5g Lovage

Directions:

Heat the pot over high heat and cook the creams in 1 tamari teaspoon and one olive oil teaspoon for 2–3 minutes. Transfer the creeping things to a plate. Wipe the pan clean with paper from the kitchen because you'll need it again.

Cook the noodles for 5–8 minutes or as directed to the packet in boiling water. Drain and reserve.

In the remaining oil, fry the garlic, chili and ginger, red onion, celery, beans, and kale for about 2-3 minutes at medium-high heat. Attach the supply and steam until it cooks the vegetables but is still crunchy, then simmer for a minute or two.

Fill the pan with creams, noodles and celery/Lovage leaves, bring back to boil, take off the heat, and serve.

Nutrition:

Calories: 288

Fat: 21.5g

Protein: 22.9g

DINNER

Salmon Sirt Super Salad

Preparation time: 10 minutes

Cooking time: 0 minutes

Servings: 1

Ingredients:

50g rocket50g chicory leaves

100g smoked salmon slices (you can also use lentils, cooked   chicken breast or tinned tuna)

80g avocado, peeled, stoned and sliced40g celery, sliced

*20g red onion, sliced 15g walnuts, chopped One tabs capers

One large Medjool date, pitted and chopped

One tabs extra-virgin olive oil Juice ¼ lemon 10g parsley, chopped

10g Lovage or celery leaves, chopped

Directions:

Arrange the leaves of the salad on a large pan. Mix all the remaining ingredients and pour over the berries.

Nutrition:

Calories: 39 Net carbs: 0.1g Fat: 1.7g Protein: 5.5g

Chapter 6 Phase Two Diet (Last 4 Days Of The Week)

Day 11 and 18

BREAKFAST

Sirtfood Breakfast Scramble

Preparation time: 10 minutes

Cooking time: 10 minutes

Servings: 1

Ingredients:

1 teaspoon mild curry powder

½ bird's eye chili, thinly sliced

2 eggs

1 teaspoon ground turmeric

Handful of thinly sliced mushrooms

5g of parsley, sliced finely

20g Kale, roughly chopped

1 tablespoon extra-virgin olive oil

Directions:

Mix the curry and turmeric powder, then apply a little water until a soft paste has been produced.

Steam up the Kale for 2–3 minutes.

And fry the chili and mushrooms for 2–3 minutes before they start browning and softening.

Add the eggs and spice paste, and cook over medium heat, then add the kale and continue cooking for another minute over medium heat. Attach the parsley, then blend well and enjoy. BBQ Tempeh Sandwiches and Baked Beans Mole

Nutrition:

Calories: 353

Net carbs: 28.1g

Fat: 9.8g

Fiber: 4.9g

Protein: 40.3g

LUNCH:

Honey, Garlic And Chili Oven-Roasted Squash

Preparation time: 10 minutes

Cooking time: 45 minutes

Servings: 4

Ingredients:

1kg assorted squash and pumpkin (at least five different types), cut in medium size pieces

3 Tablespoon olive oil3 whole garlic cloves, lightly crushed

4 red or green chilies, slit down the middle 2 sprigs thyme

3 Tablespoon (15 ml) honey 1 sprig rosemary Salt and pepper to taste

Directions:

Preheat the oven to 150 °C. Add all ingredients into a wide bowl and allow to stand for 30 minutes, mixing occasionally. In a roasting tray, place the Squash and cover with foil.

Roast covered at 150 ° C for 10 minutes.

Increase the temperature of the oven to 180 ° C, remove the foil, and roast for another 10 minutes to allow the Squash to caramel lightly

Nutrition:

Calories: 182 Net carbs: 21.5g Fat: 0.1g Protein: 1.8g

Day 12 and 19

BREAKFAST

Apple Pancakes With Blackcurrant Compote

Preparation time: 10 minutes

Cooking time: 30 minutes

Servings: 4

Ingredients:

75g porridge oats

125g plain flour

2 tablespoon caster sugar

*Pinch of salt

1 teaspoon baking powder

2 apples, peeled, cored and cut into small pieces

300ml partially skimmed milk

2 egg whites

2 teaspoon light olive oil

For the Compote

120g blackcurrants washed and stalks removed

2 tablespoon caster sugar

Directions:

Make the compote first. In a medium saucepan, placed the blackcurrants, sugar, and tea. Bring to a cooker and simmer for 10-15 minutes.

In a big pot, combine the oats, flour, baking powder, caster sugar, and salt and blend well. Stir in the apple and whisk a little at a time in the milk before you have a smooth mix. Whisk the egg whites to strong peaks, then drop the pancake into the starch. Bring the batter into a pan.

Heat 1/2 teaspoon of oil over medium-high heat in a non-stick frying pan and add approximately one-quarter of the batter. Cook until light brown, on all hands. Remove for four pancakes and repeat to produce.

Eat the pancakes drizzled over with blackcurrant compote. Sweet and Sour Tofu with brown rice

Nutrition:

Calories: 337

Net carbs: 40 g

Fat: 9.82g

Fiber: 6.2 g

Protein: 32g

LUNCH

Homemade Roasted Celery Hummus

Preparation time: 10 minutes

Cooking time: 45minutes

Servings: 1

Ingredients:

1 green serrano chili, minced (optional)

1 cup cooked chickpeas

1/3 cup tahini

2 tablespoons fresh lime or lemon juice

4 stalks of celery, trimmed and cut into 1 cm pieces (about 1 cup)

5 tablespoons olive oil (preferably EV)

2 pods of garlic

1 teaspoon salt or to taste

1 tablespoon minced parsley

Directions:

Place the celery into a baking platter.

Top with two spoonful's of oil.

Place the two garlic pods in a plate corner, and scatter with the chili.

Bake it in a 350-degree oven for 45 minutes.

Put the chickpeas into the mixer.

Carry some remaining oil into the mixer, in the hot roasted celery and other vegetables.

Add tahini, lime or lemon juice, salt, and mix until light and smooth for 3-4 minutes.

Remove from the blender into a bowl, add the remaining three tablespoons of olive oil and chopped parsley.

Nutrition:

Calories: 107

Net carbs: 7.7g

Fat: 4.5g

Fiber: 0.2g

Protein: 8.6g

DINNER

Salmon And Spinach Quiche

Preparation time: 5 minutes

Cooking time: 10 minutes

Servings: 1

Ingredients: 1 fillet of salmon 40 g mixed leaves of salad

40g green leaves of spinach2 radishes, cut and sliced thinly

2 onions of spring, trimmed and sliced

1 tiny handful parsley, chopped roughly

Directions: Preheat the oven to 180 ° C (200 ° C). Put the fillet on a baking tray and bake it 16–18 minutes before the fillet has just been cooked. Take off the oven and set aside. The salmon in the salad is equally nice hot, or cold. If the salmon is skinny, just cook the meat and separate it from the meat with a fish slice. When cooked, it should slide off easily. Combine the mayonnaise, yogurt, vinegar rice, mint leaves, and salt and pepper in a small bowl and let at least 5 minutes stand to enable the mixture to start. Place the spinach and the salad leaves and the radishes, the cucumber, the spring onions and the parsley on the serving plate. Drop the salmon on the salad and drizzle on the sauce.

Nutrition: Calories: 903 Protein: 65.28 g Fat: 59.79 g Carbohydrates: 30.79 g

Day 13 and 20

BREAKFAST

Smoked Salmon Omelets

Preparation time: 10 minutes

Cooking time: 10 minutes

Servings: 2

Ingredients:

2 Medium eggs 100g Smoked salmon, sliced 1/2 teaspoon Capers

10 g Rocket, chopped 1 teaspoon Parsley, chopped

1 teaspoon extra virgin olive oil

Directions:

In a tub, smash the eggs and whisk well. Attach the salmon, capers, peters, and fired.

In a non-stick frying pan, fire up the olive oil until heated but not burnt. Attach the mixture of the eggs and transfer the mixture around the casserole using a spatula or slice of fish before reasonable. Reduce fire, and let the omelet to cook. Slide along the sides of the spatula and roll up or split the omelet in half to eat.

Nutrition:

Calories: 471 Net carbs: 3.3g Fat: 38.72g Fiber: 1.5g Protein: 27g

LUNCH

Baked Cod Miso-Marinated With Stir Fried Green

Preparation time: 10 minutes

Cooking time: 30 minutes

Servings: 2

Ingredients:

20g) miso

One tablespoon miring

1 tablespoon extra-virgin olive oil

200g) skinless cod fillet

20g) red onion, sliced

40g) celery, sliced

Two garlic cloves, finely chopped

1 Thai chili, finely chopped

One teaspoon finely chopped fresh ginger

60g) green beans

50g) kale, roughly chopped

One teaspoon sesame seeds

5g) parsley, roughly chopped

One tablespoon tamari (or soy sauce, if not avoiding gluten)

40g) buckwheat

*One teaspoon ground turmeric

Directions:

Mix the one teaspoon of oil with the miso and mirin. Rub the cod all over, and leave for 30 minutes to marinate. Heat the oven to 220°C.

Bake the cod for about 10 minutes.

Meanwhile, bring the remaining oil to a large frying pan or wok. Stir-fry the onion for a few minutes, then incorporate the celery, garlic, chili, ginger, green beans, and kale. Toss and fry until the kale is cooked clean and soft. To help the cooking process, you might need to add a little water to the pan.

Cook the buckwheat along with the turmeric according to the packet directions.

To the stir-fry, add the sesame seeds, parsley, and tamari and serve with buckwheat and fish.

Nutrition:

Calories: 547 Net carbs: 72.7g Fat: 16.5g Fiber: 14.8g Protein: 32.1g

DINNER

Prawn Arrabbiata

Preparation time: 10 minutes

Cooking time: 40 minutes

Servings:2

Ingredients:

125-150g Raw or cooked prawns (Ideally king prawns)

65g Buckwheat pasta

1 tablespoon extra-virgin olive oil

For Arrabbiata sauce

40g Red onion, finely chopped

1 Garlic clove, finely chopped

30g Celery, finely chopped

1 Bird's eye chili, finely chopped

1 teaspoon Dried mixed herbs

1 teaspoon extra virgin olive oil

2 tablespoon White wine (optional)

400 g Tinned chopped tomatoes

1 tablespoon Chopped parsley

Directions:

Fry the onion, garlic, celery, and chili over medium-low heat and dried herbs in the oil for 1–2 minutes. Turn the heat to medium, then add the wine and cook 1 minute. Add the tomatoes and leave the sauce to cook for 20-30 minutes over medium-low heat until it has a nice rich consistency.

While the sauce is heating, bring a pan of water to the boil and cook the pasta as instructed by the packet. Drain, toss with the olive oil when cooked to your liking, and keep in the pan until needed.

Add the raw prawns to the sauce and cook for another 3–4 minutes until they have turned pink and opaque, then add the parsley and serve. If you use cooked prawns, add the parsley, bring the sauce to the boil and serve.

Add the cooked pasta to the sauce and mix properly, then heat gently.

Nutrition:

Calories: 380

Fat: 10g

Net Carbs: 44g

Fiber: 5g

Protein: 30g

Day 14 and 21

BREAKFAST

Porridge With Pineapple

Preparation time: 10 minutes

Cooking time: 10 minutes

Servings: 1

Ingredients:

70 Milliliters of oat milk 2nd Pinch of turmeric (ground)

2nd Pinch of coriander (ground)

40 Grams of millet (millet-buckwheat porridge, or oatmeal)

100 Grams of pineapple (in cubes) 1 Teaspoon rapeseed oil

50 Grams of frozen blueberries 1 Teaspoon ginger syrup

2nd Tablespoon walnuts (chopped)

Directions:

Boil 50 ml water, oat drink, spices and millet-buckwheat mixture according to the package instructions. Roast pineapple cubes in rapeseed oil. Add blueberries, ginger syrup, walnuts, arrange the porridge with the fruits.

Nutrition: Calories: 259 Net carbs: 36g Fat: 7.68g Fiber: 7.4g

Protein: 14.26g

LUNCH

Papaya Bowl With Tuna

Preparation time: 15 minutes

Cooking time: 0 minutes

Servings: 2

Ingredients:

40g of iceberg lettuce (cut) 1 Tin of tuna

140g of papaya (papaya pulp, sliced)

1 Tablespoon papaya (papaya seeds) 100g of cucumber (sliced)

0.5 red peppers (finely sliced) 2nd Tablespoons of lime juice

1 Teaspoon camelina oil Pepper (freshly ground) Salt 40g of bread

Directions:

Fill iceberg lettuce, tuna salad, papaya, papaya seeds, cucumber and bell pepper into a storage box or lunch box.

Mix lime juice, camelina oil, pepper, salt and 1-2 teaspoons of water and drizzle over the vegetables. Close the can. Pack the bread strips separately.

Nutrition:

Calories: 464 Protein: 24.23 g Fat: 37.84 g Carbohydrates: 7.33 g

LUNCH

Chicken Tagine With Fennel And Hariss Cream

Preparation time: 5 minutes

Cooking time: 30 minutes

Servings: 2

Ingredients:

40g of whole grain rice

80g of chicken (see recipe "Chicken Tagine with Fennel")

2nd Spring onions (in rings)

1 Carrot (grated)

150g of pineapple (in pieces)

150g of red cabbage (finely sliced)

2nd Tablespoon apple cider vinegar

1 Tablespoons orange jam (bitter)

3rd Tablespoons of orange juice

3rd Tablespoons chicken broth (bouillon)

1 TL curry powder (medium hot)

Cayenne pepper

5 Teaspoon linseed oil (or rapeseed oil)

Salt

2nd Tablespoon cashew nuts (roasted)

Directions:

Mix the rice, chicken, spring onions, carrot, pineapple and red cabbage loosely.

Mix together apple cider vinegar, jam, orange juice, stock, curry and cayenne pepper. Fold in linseed oil with a fork and mix the dressing with the rice salad and season with salt.

Divide the salad into 2 portions. Put one half in a glass and arrange the other half on a plate. Chill the salad in a glass and eat the next day.

Nutrition:

Calories: 381

Net carbs: 4.1g

Fat: 27.7g

Fiber: 0.6g

Protein: 27.6g:

DINNER

Tortilla With Herb Tomatoes

Preparation time: 10 minutes

Cooking time: 35 minutes

Servings: 4

Ingredients:

180g of chili pepper (green, or 1 green bell pepper, in thin slices)

2nd red onion (in rings)

250g of mushrooms (sliced)

1 Tablespoons of rapeseed oil

60g of smoked tofu (finely chopped)

1 Tablespoons of thyme leaves

Pepper (freshly ground)

Seasoned Salt

Oil (baking oil for the mold)

5 Organic eggs (size M)

5 Tablespoons milk

1 Clove of garlic (crushed)

100g of tomato (chopped)

2nd Tablespoons herbal mixture (fresh or frozen, chopped)

Directions:

Preheat the oven to 180 degrees.

Braise the peppers, onions and mushrooms in rapeseed oil for 3-4 minutes. Mix in the smoked tofu and thyme. Pepper vigorously and salt a little. Spray a rectangular, ovenproof dish (26 x 4 x 17 cm) with baking oil. Lightly whisk eggs, milk and garlic. Mix egg mass and vegetables and pour everything into the mold and smooth out. Bake the tortilla in the oven for 25 minutes.

Mix tomatoes with herb salt and herbs. Take out the tortilla, let it cool slightly, cut half into cubes and arrange herb tomatoes with half.

Nutrition:

Calories: 425

Net carbs: 0.5g

Fat: 5.9g

Protein: 22.8g

Chapter 7 What Do I Do After The Diet? How To "Sirtify" Your Lifestyle

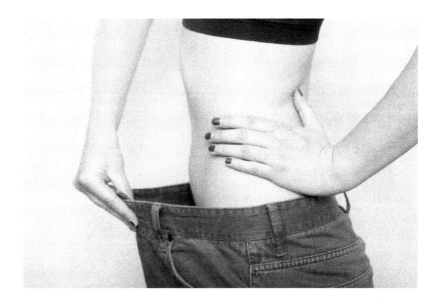

The greatest thing about the Sirtfood diet is that is not a diet! It's a change in lifestyle, so how can you implement it after the three weeks of "diet" that have boosted your metabolism and supercharged your energy levels?

Return to three meals a day:

During Phase 1 you consumed just one or two meals a day, which gave you lots of flexibility over when you ate your meals, but now that you are returning to "normal" habits, you should really be mindful of your breakfast. Eating a healthy, balanced breakfast increases our energy and concentration levels. A number of studies shows that people who regularly eat breakfast are less likely to be overweight.

This high levels of energies are achieved not only by eating a Sirtfood-rich breakfast, but especially through the inclusion of the green juice, which you should have either first thing in the morning—at least thirty minutes before breakfast —or midmorning. Many people who drink their green juice first thing and do not feel hungry for a couple of hours afterward. If this is the effect it has on you, it is perfectly fine to wait a couple of hours before having breakfast. Just don't skip it. Alternatively, you can kick off your day with a good breakfast, then wait two or three hours before having the green juice. Be flexible and just go with whatever works for you.

What about snacking?

Snacks have been branded as the devil incarnate. "To lose weight you have to give up snacks", how many times have you heard it?

It's not true, if you have had a busy day and you're rushing between work, home, and getting around with kids, it's perfectly normal to need something to tide you over between meals. You can enjoy some guilt-free treats made entirely out of Sirtfoods!

"Sirtifying" your meals

The thinking goes if it's just for three weeks, I can eat anything… But this shouldn't be the case with the Sirtfood diet. You shouldn't worry constantly about food restrictions, just take a look at the recipe and you will realize that they are clever, tasty twists on classics. So, they will be easy to incorporate in your life and the life of those around you, be it children or fussy hosts. Examples include the delicious Sirtfood smoothie for the perfect on-the-go breakfast, and the simple switch from wheat to buckwheat for adding extra taste and zip to what seemed the guilty-pleasure of pasta. Meanwhile iconic, beloved dishes such as chili con carne and curry don't even need much change, with the traditional recipes offering Sirtfood goodness. And who said fast food meant bad food? Find the authentic vibrant flavors of a pizza and remove the guilt by making it yourself. There's no need to say farewell to indulgence either, as proven by our pancakes laden with berries and dark chocolate sauce. It's not even dessert, its breakfast, and it's great for you. Simple changes: you continue to eat the foods you love while driving a healthy weight and well-being. And that is the dietary revolution that is Sirtfoods.

Don't stick to just the top 20 sirtfoods

The top 20 sirtfoods are great sources of SIRT-activating ingredients, but that doesn't mean that you should only eat those for the rest of your life. There are other ingredients that are healthy and have analogue SIRT-activating functions. Goggins and Mattens have only picked out the best of the best. But feel free to expand your diet, actually you are encouraged to do it to achieve a more balanced lifestyle and a continued wellbeing.

How about proteins?

Proteins are a staple of the Sirtfood diet, as you will see in the recipes. You can consume eggs, dairy, poultry, and red meat. Just stay away from processed meat, or at least reduce their consumption significantly. Vegans should be mindful of integrating iodine, calcium, and vitamin B12, but that is true for any diet.

Tips for cooking with Sirtfoods:

When trying to cook with the sirtfoods most of the ingredients you should be familiar with already. However, there are a few which will be new.

Matcha is green tea, but in a powdered form. You're unlikely to be able to buy it from the shelves of your local supermarket, but it will be available from health specialist stores or from online retailers. Matcha is generally produced in China and Japan, where it is a traditional beverage, so you should expect to order from overseas.

It is better if you can buy Matcha from Japan, as Matcha from China may have forms of pollution and impurities due to the environment. Matcha green tea is used in Zen ceremonies in Japan and it is even better for you than regular green tea. The unique nature of Matcha green tea originates from how it is grown. Matcha is grown almost entirely in dark shadowy environments, whilst green tea is usually grown in bright sunshine.

Matcha is also ground into a power using a mill, rather than being cut into small leaves and added as an infusion.

Chapter 8 Essential Foods In A Sirt Diet

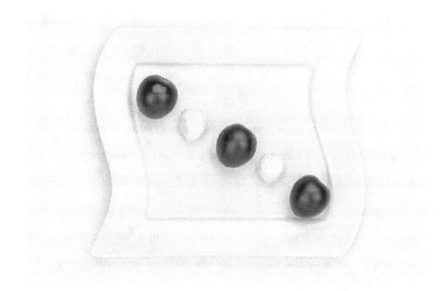

T he high protein sources, along with the top twenty foods in the sirtfood diet, are an essential combination. In the first week of the diet, it is essential that you will consume nearly 1000 calories per day. If this calorie deficit diet is loaded with proteins, essential fats, and low glycemic carbohydrates, you will decrease plenty of extra body fat in no time. Here is a bonus of using the sirtfood diet with a high protein combo. You will lose a significant proportion of extra body fat, and you will also have a high possibility of gaining several pounds of lean muscle mass. There is a question, is an increase in lean muscle mass dangerous? The question is tricky and has a great answer. The answer is "No." an increase in lean muscle mass while decreasing the fat percentage is absolutely a win-win. The reason behind this is the possibility of getting more fit while decreasing the risks of many illnesses associated with high body fat percentages.

How is an increase in lean muscle mass safe?

The reason is pretty apparent. If you increase your lean muscle mass, you will get the buffed physique, and the chances of getting diseases associated with gain fat will be reduced comparatively. But if someone wants to stick to a specific body-mass index ratio, he may find increasing total lean muscle mass a bit of a problem. We will discuss in detail how BMI is not a real source of measuring the fitness of a body and how it has lost its spot of being a gold standard for a very long time. If someone is trying to put up some weight because he is skinny, he has to consume more than he burns. Let's say he burns 1500 calories daily, so to gain weight, he should eat a minimum of 1750 calories daily. Those 150 extra calories will put some safe weight in his body. But what if he consumes 1750 calories daily from high saturated and Tran's fat sources along with plenty of carbohydrates? Here is a big problem. He will plainly put up some weight but with extra fat and low lean muscle mass. So, he can be successful in his primary goal of gaining weight, but he is at high risk of getting diseases like obesity, heart attack, diabetes, and fatty liver. Moreover, losing that extra fat is also a hard nut to crack.

So, what if he consumes 1750 calories daily through high protein sources, well-balanced fats, and good carbohydrates? Of course, he is winning over millions because he is investing very right in his body to achieve his goals. He will gain weight but lean muscle mass only due to high protein and a balanced diet. His overall body fat percentage will be lowered, and his body will be more muscular. Moreover, he will reduce fat from his viscera such as liver and stomach, and chances of getting diseases associated with obesity will be lowered too much extent.

In the second scenario, if a person wants to lose weight, he has to consume less than he burns. If he burns 1500 calories daily, he should consume less than 1500 calories daily. Let say he starts by consuming 1000 calories daily, but from carbohydrates and bad fats, he is making a big mistake. His weight will drop for initial 5-7 days; then, his body will undergo an emergency response to put up the weight by converting protein and carbohydrates into fats and storing them in the body. It is the worst case because he will end up with plenty of extra fat rather than decreasing it, and his calorie deficit diet will bring no benefit to him. So, in that case, he must be losing his energy as well as an overall sense of well-being. But if he consumes the same 1000 calories from a high protein source and balanced amounts of fats and carbs, he will be losing plenty of fats along with gaining lean muscle mass. So it is actually a win-win situation.

Body-mass index (BMI) is not perfect:

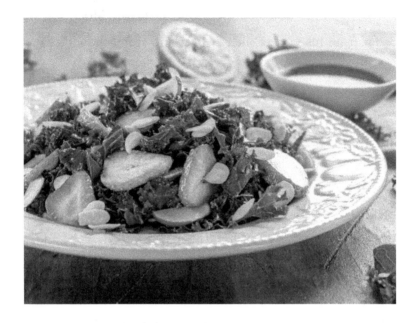

For a very long time, fitness experts and doctors are using BMI as the most valid source of checking the obesity levels in a body. It is achieved by measuring the height and weight of a person, and a standard is maintained throughout different age groups to check the levels of obesity or underweight categories. However, we put you through a scenario in which you will find it hard to defend this position of BMI as a gold standard of obesity. If let's say a person is 18 years old and he has a body fat percentage of 35% with BMI 23, can you categories him fit? According to BMI, 18-25 is the safe limit, and above 25 will be categories as obese. So, he is not obese in that case, right? Let's dig in to find the truth. So, that male person has 25% extra fat on his body, but because he doesn't have more lean muscle mass, his weight is in BMI safe limit. But he actually has a lot of extra fat. So, what should we do now? The answer is, don't listen to BMI because it is now well established that BMI is failed in this scenario

Professionals are not using BMI for many decades, but we don't know why it still has its hype in society. In the above example, an obese person can easily be categorized as safe according to BMI. 35% of body fat is too much, and his low lean muscle mass is another thorny issue. This person is at high risk of getting severe obesity-related illnesses like stroke, heart attack, and diabetes. In another scenario, a person of the same age and same weight with the same BMI has 8%v total body fat. You can consider him absolutely fit because he got the right weight with plenty of lean muscle mass and a meager body fat percentage. Everyone should follow this physique goal.

Another turning point related to BMI is its wrong perception of obesity. In another scenario, a person has 8% body fat with the same height and age, but his BMI is 29. Is he obese, right? No, he is not obese just because of higher BMI. He may be a pro weight lifter or bodybuilder who has vast lean muscle mass with a very low-fat percentage, but his weight is above the borderline of obesity as calculated by BMI. He is not obese, and he got more protein on his body, which is very safe because he has deficient body fat. But BMI will mark him obese. So, now you can say that BMI is not actually the correct marker of obesity. It is the body fat percentage who will decide who is obese, underweight, or fit.

So the sirtfood diet helps you gaining more lean muscle mass and losing more fat, making you fitter and healthier.

A detailed discussion on Macro and micronutrients:

If you want to master the science of the sirtfood diet, you should know all the necessary components from which our diet is made. There are two broad categories of nutrients, which are called the macro and micronutrients. Let's discuss these nutrients in detail:

Macro-nutrients:

As the name implies, macronutrients are the essential nutrients that comprise a more significant portion of our daily diet. These are essential because they form the foundation of daily caloric intake, and these are rich in energy. Macronutrients are three in types:

1. Protein

2. Fats

3. Carbohydrates

Protein: protein is the most critical type of macronutrient. The most important sources of protein are Whey protein isolates, Casein protein, Salmon, Tuna, Chicken, Turkey, Beef, Mutton, Dairy, Egg white, and some fruits/vegetables as well. A diet which comprises of high levels of protein can provide more advantage of getting lean muscle mass over those diets which lack sufficient amounts of protein. Protein is also an essential precursor of our enzymes, and our blood also has some essential types of proteins. So, having a high protein regime along with the sirtfood diet is a successful idea to get a ripped physique as well as low body fat.

Fats: Fats are also called lipids and are essential energy supplies for the human body. Fats contain nine calories per gram, which are more than double the protein and carbohydrates (4 calories per gram). This is the reason that body naturally stores fats as an emergency supply when we undergo a calorie deficit dieting. The most significant benefit of storing fat as an emergency supply is it's hard to break and easy to consume characteristic. Adipose tissues are hard to break, and thus, they are an excellent source of energy supply for the crisis. There are different classifications of fats. Mono and polyunsaturated fatty acids are the highest quality fatty acids that are present in olive oils, some other plant oils, and some fish oils. Saturated fats are also essential to consume because of our hormones; mostly, the sex hormones are based on saturated fatty acids which can be found in some animal and plant basis. The worst and never to consume the type of fatty acids are trans-fatty acids, which are needed to avoid because of very harmful effects in our bodies.

A well-balanced diet should have fats in 0.5 grams per pound of bodyweight proportion, and zero consumption of any fat as achieved in some inferior yet trendy fat loss diets should be avoided because of severe health risks.

Carbohydrates: carbohydrates are also termed as sugars, and the most consumed type of macronutrients around the globe are actually the carbs. Carbohydrates can be low, medium, and high glycemic. Some carbs are simple, yet others are complex. A diet must have low and medium glycemic carbs such as oatmeal, honey, and fruits, but carbs having high glycemic indexes such as processed sugars and soda should be avoided. High glycemic carbs cause a rapid spike in blood sugar levels, and thus, it can lead to diabetes. However, complex high glycemic carbs can be utilized post-workout because they are essential to replenish the burnt glycogen storage in a human body after exercise.

Carbohydrates are those macronutrients that can be cycled, and the calorie deficit cyclic diet should per iodize the carbohydrate intake to get maximum results with minimum leptin production and long-lasting results. Luckily, the sirtfood diet is well designed to provide all the essential carbs, yet cycling them in this diet provides rapid and long-lasting fat loss in a short duration of time.

Micro-nutrients: this category of nutrients in our daily diet comprises of those salts, minerals, and vitamins which are present in food inherently, or we can take them as a supplement. Iron, magnesium, calcium, potassium, and vitamins are some examples. Some of them are required in trace amounts, yet they are essential for the proper regulation of the body's essential cycles.

So this is the end of this critical discussion. Everyone who intends to follow the sirtfood diet should know all these factors to formulate their own customized diet plan rather than following a copy-pasted well for all content.

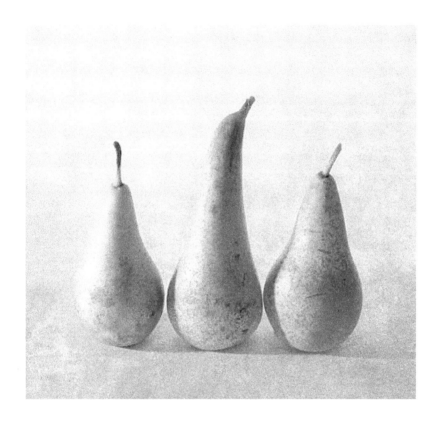

Chapter 9 Sirtuin Facts And Fiction

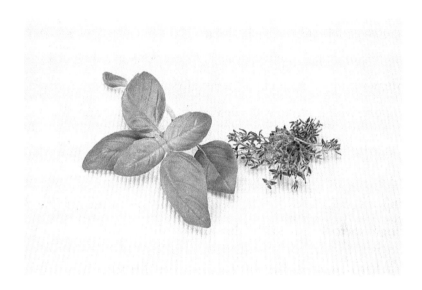

Build Muscle

Sirtuins are genes that activate proteins in your body. Protein is a very popular word in the world of fitness and we all know that it is absolutely necessary for building the strong muscles that you see gracing the covers of fitness magazines. But protein is far more important than simply developing bulky muscle mass. Protein is the building block of every single cell in your body.

We all need protein to survive, let alone thrive and look youthful and strong.

Yes, a body that has only lean fat and nicely toned muscles will create an aesthetically pleasing, athletic picture. But muscle is also responsible for holding our skeletons in place, preventing bone loss and joint damage, and keeping our vital organs protected and safe. In fact, our most vital organ, our heart, is a muscle. Just as our muscle protects everything inside our skin, proteins also protect everything inside our cells. Sirtuins insulate our cells and protect them from the damage that a stressful, toxic environment cause. Our bodies are designed to keep us safe, with many different systems of defense in order, but we need to support these systems with the nutrition we consume.

Unfortunately, many of us are starting from a position of current ill-health and probably have a certain amount of excess weight that is causing us difficulty. Muscle and protein are some of the most important factors of shedding that extra body fat.

Muscle has a much harder job than fat does. Muscle is what allows us to move constantly throughout the day, even if it is just our heart beating. Fat, on the other hand, is designed to simply remain in our bodies, inactive and lazy, until it is needed as an emergency supply of energy. It's not difficult to understand, then, that muscle is going to require a lot more energy to maintain itself.

The more muscle you have in your body, the more energy you will burn in a day. This will not only build a strong, healthy body, but it will also accelerate weight loss and promote healthy weight management in the long-term.

Diets that focus exclusively on calorie restriction will force your body to use any energy it finds and, for a period of time, you will lose weight. That weight will come from a variety of sources, including fat, muscle and water. If you reach your goal weight, or if you simply return to your normal calorie consumption, your body will refill all the reserves you just emptied, putting all the weight right back on your body.

With the Sirtfood Diet, calorie restriction is limited to a single week, simply to give your body a chance to empty out some of the overwhelming food your metabolic system is coping with. After that first week, you will instead be prioritizing the addition of foods that help to activate protein and build healthy muscle cells. This will provide the perfect foundation for complete cellular health, and it will maximize your weight loss efforts until your body naturally returns to its ideal composition.

In the original pilot study during the development stages of the Sirtfood Diet, participants had every morsel of food prepared for them to ensure compliance and their body composition was monitored every step of the way. It quickly became obvious that, even though the average weight loss was slightly more than 5 pounds in the first week of the diet, muscle mass was not only maintained, but it increased by 1 – 2 pounds.

For those of you who are cringing at the idea of adding any amount of weight to your body, you should realize that muscle, in addition to burning more energy, also takes up less space than fat. This means that if you were to lose 2 pounds of fat and gain 2 pounds of muscle, though the number on the scale will be the same, your body will be physically smaller which, after all, is the primary goal. In regard to the pilot study, if the weight loss was adjusted to reflect muscle gain, the average would be increased to approximately 7 pounds within a single week (Goggins & Matten, 2018).

The scientific reasoning for this extraordinary result is the activation of your sirtuin genes, which guard your cells against protein loss and muscle breakdown. As long as we're activating our sirtuins, even in a caloric deficit, our muscles will be protected and working in our favor. Without the activation of sirtuins, our muscles will actually shrink because they don't have the ability to develop or regenerate when damaged.

It isn't just the size or quantity of muscle that you have in your body that is important, but it is also the biological age of those muscles. One of the cruel realities of growing older is that damage in our body accumulates over the years, resulting in what we commonly see as age-related health decline. While all bodies will sustain some levels of damage simply by being alive and exposed to countless varieties of stress, there are ways to mitigate the damage and keep your cells biologically more youthful than you might be chronologically. Sirtuins are very effective at keeping your muscles young, despite your age.

When you follow the Sirtfood Diet, you will be providing your body with everything it needs to protect against the damage that stress causes. Your cells will be better equipped to fight off free radicals and recover from chronic inflammation, which are both known to be root factors in stress and many other chronic diseases. If we can protect our muscle mass, we will also inherently be protecting our bodies against the ravages of age.

The more you protect and develop healthy muscles, the healthier you will be overall and the easier it will be to find and stay at your ideal body weight. Sirtuins, activated by sirtfoods, are the easiest, most effective and delicious way to accomplish this.

Burn Fat

In addition to protecting your muscles, sirtfoods encourage your metabolic system to start burning through the fat that is stored in your body, which is one of the reasons for the surprising weight loss potential.

Gaining weight is a complex process for humans that involves multiple hormones sending signals back and forth to your various biological processes. One of these hormones, insulin, I'm sure you're familiar with.

When you consume any calories, your body needs to convert the food into glucose so that it can be used as energy to keep your body functioning. Some foods, such as sugar or refined carbohydrates, for example, convert to sugar in your bloodstream almost instantaneously, causing a spike in blood glucose levels.

Other foods, like complex carbohydrates and proteins, take longer for your body to break down and convert to glucose, so your blood gets a slower and steady drip of glucose.

When your blood sugar gets too high because you've consumed more sugar than your body needs to operate immediately, it can cause a variety of problems. Headaches, thirst or fatigue might be experienced in the short-term, but high blood sugar levels can lead to kidney failure, heart disease or nerve damage if the issue becomes chronic.

Obviously, these symptoms are severe and potentially life-threatening, so your body has a process to detect high blood sugar levels and bring them back down: it releases insulin.

With the help of your liver and cholesterol, insulin pulls sugar out of your bloodstream and tells your cells to take it in instead and your blood glucose levels drop as your fat cells get a little fuller.

When your blood sugar gets too low, another hormone, glucagon, will be released. Glucagon taps your liver and fat cells in order to release the stored glucose back into your bloodstream.

The main problem with our modern diet is that humans have developed the habit of constant grazing and/or over-eating. This provides a constant flow of glucose, triggering a constant need for insulin. Our blood sugar rarely dips low enough to trigger the production of glucagon, so instead of using our stored energy, we simply add more to the reserves.

Swapping a Standard American Diet (SAD) that causes an instant spike in your blood glucose for a Sirtfood Diet, which will create a slower and steady flow of energy will help to reinstate that natural balance of hormones once again. As an added bonus, studies have shown that activating sirtuins can actually suppress your body's ability to store fat as it increases the propensity to burn it (Picard, et al., 2004). Your metabolic system will actually have a chance to use the stored energy.

Aside from sirtfoods being a more balancing form of energy, by activating our sirtuin genes our cells are being protected and fortified. Each cell has a power center called a mitochondrion which is responsible for the conversion of glucose into useable energy. This is a lot of work for our cells and, especially if we are eating more calories than we need and those calories are primarily simple carbohydrates, our mitochondria wear out quickly.

Sirtuins protect our mitochondria, allowing them to process energy more efficiently. In other words, we can burn fat more quickly.

Sirtfoods work on multiple fronts to help our body naturally regulate weight: they reduce the amount of glucose that gets stored as fat, and they increase the speed at which our fat gets used.

As an added bonus, by naturally regulating our metabolism, we can protect ourselves against insulin resistance and type 2 diabetes.

Insulin and glycogen aren't the only hormones to return to a healthy balance on a Sirtfood Diet. Leptin is also regulated.

Leptin resistance isn't as commonly understood as insulin resistance, but it plays just as important of a role in the process of weight gain. Leptin is often called the hunger hormone because it's responsible for telling your brain when you have enough fat stored in your body to keep you safe, and when you need to take in more energy.

If you have low body fat, your brain will throw out hunger signals to encourage you to eat more food. Unfortunately, if you have damaged leptin receptors, your brain will also continue to pump out hunger signals, whether you're actually in need of energy or not.

Hunger is very hard to ignore, and if your leptin levels are dysregulated, not only are you going to feel hungry constantly, but your body will also be actively trying to store any energy you consume as fat instead of using it immediately.

When you follow a Sirtfood Diet, your leptin levels will naturally balance and your hunger signals will only start to spark when you truly need more nutrition. Not simply when your sugar crash has taken a turn for the worse.

Chapter 10 Benefits Of Sirtfood Diet

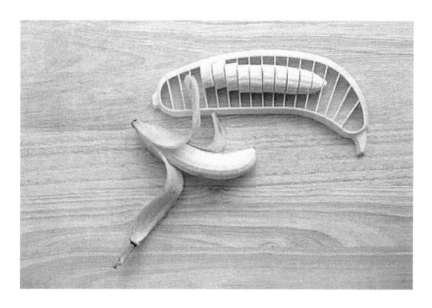

What are the advantages?

Y ou will get more fit on the off chance that you follow this eating regimen intently. "Regardless of whether you're eating 1,000 calories of tacos, 1,000 calories of kale, or 1,000 calories of snickerdoodles, you will get more fit at 1,000 calories!" says Dr. Youdim. In any case, she additionally brings up that you can have accomplishment with a progressively sensible calorie limitation. The run of the mill every day caloric admission of somebody not on an eating routine is 2,000 to 2,200, so decreasing to 1,500 is as yet confining and would be a successful weight reduction procedure for most, she says.

Are there any safety measures?

This arrangement is severe with little squirm room or substitutions, and weight reduction must be kept up if the low caloric admission is likewise kept up, making it hard to hold fast to the long haul. That implies any weight you lost in the initial seven days is probably going to be recovered after you finish, says Dr. Youdin. Her primary concern? "Constraining protein admission with juices will bring about lost bulk. Losing muscle is synonymous with dropping your metabolic rate or 'digestion,' making weight upkeep increasingly troublesome," she says.

What do practical nourishment specialists need to state about it?

Generally speaking, master input on the Sirtfood Diet is blended. The uplifting news: The eating regimen seems to be stacked with sound nourishments. "There is broad research that features the numerous advantages of a portion of the nourishments got down on about this eating routine, similar to espresso, green tea, dull chocolate, and dim verdant greens," says Jessica Cording, R.D., enrolled dietitian and wellbeing mentor.

Vast numbers of these nourishments may likewise bolster substantial weight reduction, says Frances Large man-Roth, R.D., however, whether they advance weight reduction by actuating sirtuins stays to be demonstrated. "The nourishments advanced on the eating routine are ones that battle aggravation and would be valuable for anybody to add to their eating regimen yet not because they help sirtuins," she says. "Because nourishment contains a specific supplement connected to digestion doesn't imply that nourishment causes programmed weight reduction—it is doubtful to turn on a 'thin quality' with nourishment." Moreover, while these "sirtfoods" are without a doubt substantial, large man-Roth says somebody would need to ensure they're additionally balancing their suppers with sound fats and proteins.

Concerning the structure of the eating routine, it may not be significant. However, Cording figures it could be an agreeable choice for individuals who are keen on a weight-reduction plan that has some structure and offers space for adaptability and customization. "I welcome that it's a 'diet of incorporation' versus one concentrated basically on limiting nourishments," she says. So, Cording concedes that the juice-substantial beginning piece of Phase One is a bit lower in calories than what she'd regularly prescribe. Yet, the later stages, which incorporate a more unhealthy objective and healthy nourishment, are, to some degree, increasingly economical.

Lovage is another ingredient you probably have never heard of. Lovage is an herb, but one that hasn't been used by our culinary society for over 100 years. It can be bought, but it is more practical to grow your own. Lovage plants are low maintenance – you should be able to plant the seeds in a regular pot, put it on the windowsill in your house, water it once a day and see growth in a few weeks. Lovage seeds will be available from most garden centers (or you can buy an already thriving plant).

Additionally, you may or may not have heard of buckwheat. Buckwheat is a grain that is high in protein, carbohydrate and sirtuin. However, other foods made from buckwheat, such as buckwheat pasta or soba noodles will need to either be bought online or sourced from a specialist store.

Small variations to the main meal recipes provided can help make them more palatable. For example, Bird's-eye or Thai Chilies are more potent than the chilies typically used in the Western diet. Owing to this if you are not well-acquainted with spicy foods; you should reduce the amount you add into your recipes to begin with. Try half the recommended value, ensuring you de-seed the chili as the seeds themselves are rather spicy.

Miso is a type of soya-bean paste, which is used for flavoring in eastern dishes. Miso comes in multiple flavors, with the lighter colored variants being sweeter than the darker colors. You can experiment with what flavor suits you best. On a similar vein, the potency of the miso varies between the different colors (white, yellow, red & brown), so you might want to lower or increase the amount of miso you use to get the taste just right.

Buckwheat should be washed before it is cooked, by placing it in a sieve and rinsing it with water. Flat leaf parsley is preferable to curly leaf, but the latter is acceptable if you cannot source the former.

Finally, feel free to season and add salt and pepper as necessary, although the recipes are intended to be tasty without additional flavoring.

Now that you have all the relevant information about the Sirtfood diet and how to change to healthy, balanced lifestyle without giving up your guilty pleasures, how about we get to the good stuff? Let's take a look at the Sirtfood recipes that will change your life. I have compiled the most comprehensive Sirtfood cookbook you will find on the market!

Chapter 11 The Procedure Of The Sirtfood Diet

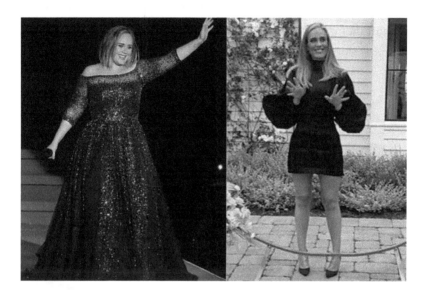

One step at a time! That's what it takes to incorporate sirtfood into your diet. The diet is simple and easy to follow in a sense that it only calls for a few definite steps to take. Firstly, you will need to increase food consumption that is rich in sirtuin, then you will have to follow the phases of the diet plus you will need to add green juices to your daily diet. Here are a couple of steps that must be followed to achieve your weight loss goals on a sirtfood diet:

1. Get the right ingredients

Remember that all this diet asks from you is to increase your sirtuins intake. That can be done only through careful and selective grocery shopping. Prepare a list of the ingredients that contain a high amount of sirtuins and check their utility as per your meal plan. There are certain ingredients like coffee, parsley, red wine, and chocolate, that you can have all the time. So, stock up your kitchen cabinets with these ingredients.

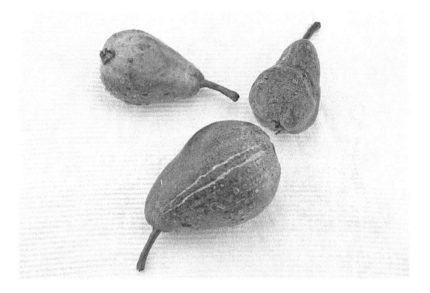

2. Set up the schedule

The sirtfood diet gives you small weight loss targets for each week. In the initial time period, you must prepare a schedule to keep track of your meals, the caloric intake, and the timing of green juices you are consuming in a day. In this way, you will be able to manage the first few days of the diet adoption easily and continue observing body changes and measure your weight to keep track of your pace.

Prepare for the first week

In the first week of the sirtfood diet, the dieter must control his caloric intake. Therefore, to avoid any mistakes or confusion, all the high caloric food items should be removed from sight. Stuff your refrigerator only with the food that is appropriate for the sirtfood diet, and keep the juices, fruits, and vegetables ready to use. Instead of planning your meal every other day, make plans for the entire week according to the caloric limitations.

3. Caloric intake

Keep in mind that sirtfood is more about weight loss, so mere sirtuins cannot magically work overnight if you keep consuming more calories than your body can actually burn. Do the math and understand your caloric needs, even when the diet does not restrict you from high caloric intake after the first seven days. Still, you must maintain a strict check on the daily caloric intake to keep the weight in control. Otherwise, it does not take much to regain the lost pounds.

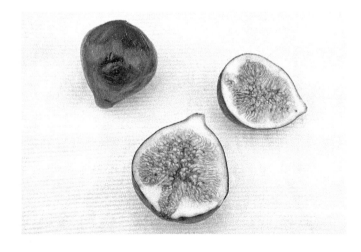

4. Green juices

Green juices are one of the most essential parts of the sirtfood diet. These are your way to detoxification and quick weight loss. Green veggies are full of phytonutrients, minerals, and antioxidants. Having them frequently throughout the day can help boost the metabolism, remove the metabolic waste from the body, and enables the body to metabolize the needed nutrients appropriately. These juices are also great for keeping electrolyte balance in the body.

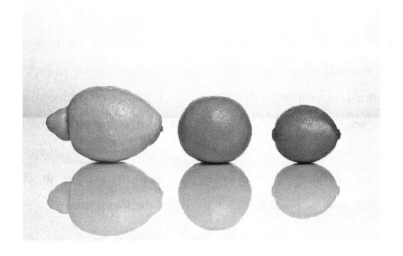

5. Maintenance

To harness the benefit of this diet or any other diet for that matter, it is imperative to maintain your new dietary routine. Most people abandon the diet as soon as they are an oven with the first two phases of the diet or when they achieve their weight loss goals. And soon, they regain weight and blame the diet for being ineffective, which is far from true. It all depends on how consistently you follow this diet plan.

Chapter 12 How To Build A Diet That Works

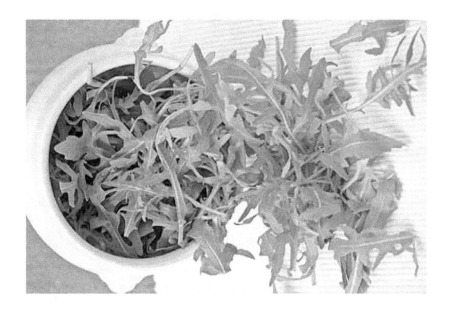

The basis of the sirtuin diet can be explained in simple terms or in complex ways. It is important to understand how and why it works however, so that you can appreciate the value of what you are doing. It is important also to know why these sirtuin rich foods help to help you maintain fidelity to your diet plan. Otherwise, you may throw something in your meal with less nutrition that would defeat the purpose of planning for one rich in sirtuins. Most importantly, this is not a dietary fad, and as you will see, there is much wisdom contained in how humans have used natural foods even for medicinal purposes, over thousands of years.

To understand how the Sirtfood diet works, and why these particular foods are necessary, we will look at the role they play in the human body.

Sirtuin activity was first researched in yeast, where a mutation caused an extension in the yeast's lifespan. Sirtuins were also shown to slow aging in laboratory mice, fruit flies, and nematodes. As research on Sirtuins proved to transfer to mammals, they were examined for their use in diet and slowing the aging process. The sirtuins in humans are different in the typing but they essentially work in the same ways and reasons.

There are seven "members" that make up the sirtuin family. It is believed that sirtuins play a big role in regulating certain functions of cells including proliferation (reproduction and growth of cells), apoptosis (death of cells). They promote survival and resist stress to increase longevity.

They are also seen to block neurodegeneration (loss or function of the nerve cells in the brain). They conduct their housekeeping functions by cleaning out toxic proteins and supporting the brain's ability to change and adapt to different conditions, or to recuperate (i.e., brain plasticity). As part of this they also help reduce chronic inflammation, and reduce something called oxidative stress. Oxidative stress is when there are too many cell-damaging free radicals circulating in the body, and the body cannot catch up by combating them with anti-oxidants. These factors are related to age-related illness and weight as well, which again, brings us back to a discussion of how they actually work.

You will see labels in Sirtuins that start with "SIR," which represents "Silence Information Regulator" genes. They do exactly that, silence or regulate, as part of their functions. The seven sirtuins that humans work with are: SIRT1, SIRT2, SIRT3, SIRT4, SIRT 5, SIRT6 and SIRT7. Each of these types is responsible for different areas of protecting cells. They work by either stimulating or turning on certain gene expressions, or by reducing and turning off other gene expressions. This essentially means that they can influence genes to do more or less of something, most of which they are already programmed to do.

Through enzyme reactions, each of the SIRT types affect different areas of cells that are responsible for the metabolic processes that help to maintain life. This is also related to what organs and functions they will affect.

For example, the SIRT6 causes an expression of genes in humans that affect skeletal muscle, fat tissue, brain, and heart. SIRT 3 would cause an expression of genes that affect the kidneys, liver, brain and heart.

If we tie these concepts together, you can see that the Sirtuin proteins can change the expression of genes, and in the case of the Sirtfood diet we care about how sirtuins can turn off those genes that are responsible for speeding up aging and for weight management.

The other aspect to this conversation of sirtuins is the function and the power of calorie restriction on the human body. Calorie restriction is simply eating less calories. This, coupled with exercise and reducing stress is usually a combination for weight loss. Calorie restriction has also proven across much research in animals and humans to increase one's lifespan.

We can look further at the role of sirtuins with calorie restriction, and using the SIRT3 protein which has a role in metabolism and aging. Amongst all of the effects of the protein on gene expression, (such as preventing cells from dying, reducing tumors from growing, etc.), we want to understand the effects of SIRT3 on weight for the purpose of this book.

The SIRT3 has high expression in those metabolically active tissues as we stated earlier, and its ability to express itself increases with caloric restriction, fasting, and exercise. On the contrary, it will express itself less when the body has a high fat, high calorie-riddled diet.

The last few highlights of sirtuins are their role in regulating telomeres and reducing inflammation which also help with staving off disease and aging.

Telomeres are sequences of proteins at the ends of chromosomes. When cells divide these get shorter. As we age they get shorter, and other stressors to the body also will contribute to this. Maintaining these longer telomeres is the key to slower aging. In addition, proper diet, along with exercise and other variables can lengthen telomeres. SIRT6 is one of the sirtuins that, if activated, can help with DNA damage, inflammation and oxidative stress. SIRT1 also helps with inflammatory response cycles that are related to many age-related diseases.

Since this, as well as fasting, is a stressor, these factors will stimulate the SIRT3 proteins to kick in and protect the body from the stressors and excess free radicals. Again, the telomere length is affected as well.

To sum up, all of this information also shows that, contrary to some people's beliefs that in terms of genetics, such as "it is what it is" or "it is my fate because Uncle Joe has something…" through our own lifestyle choices, and what we are exposed to, we can influence action and changes in our genes. This is quite an empowering thought, and yet another reason why you should be excited to have a science-based diet such as the Sirtfood diet, available to you.

Having laid this all out before you, you should be able to appreciate how and why these miraculous compounds work in your favor, to keep you youthful, healthy, and lean If they are working hard for you, don't you feel that you should do something too? Well, you can, and that is what the rest of this book will do for you.

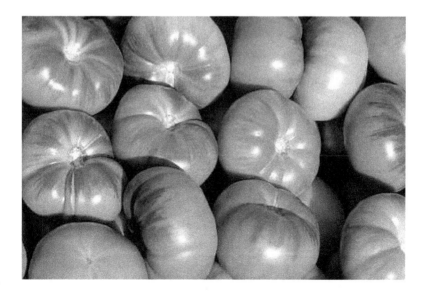

Chapter 13 Top Sirtfoods: 20 Foods That Activate Weight Loss

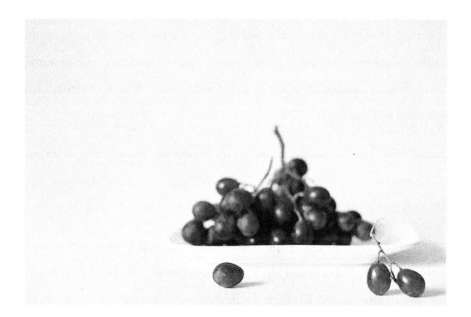

The Super Sirtfood Selection

The heart of this diet is of course the food selection. Sirtuin activators are all found in plants, but you have to take note that not all veggies and fruits have the necessary compound to consider it as Sirtfood. Examples of this non-sirtuin activator food are avocados (very popular in the world of losing weight), cucumber, bananas and carrots, although it doesn't mean that these type of fruits and veggies are not packed with benefits or not worth eating. But for our purpose, which is to tap on our body's sirtuin, you have to make sure that you will follow the list (and research more) and include it in your daily diet.

Green tea (preferable matcha powder) - A better alternative than your builder's tea is green tea. Green tea is made from steamed fresh leaves from the plant instead of the fermented leaves. This sirtuin-filled beverage is actually a popular choice for health buffs, making it the world's most consumed beverage after water. Some of the essential vitamins and minerals it contains are folate, vitamin B, magnesium and other antioxidants.

Dark Chocolate - Not just any kind of chocolate (but equally satisfying and has lower fat and sugar content), your choice should have at least 85% cocoa solids in order to be considered as Sirtfood.

Kale - This is a popular "superfood" since it is filled with antioxidants (beta-carotene, kaempferol, quercetin and more). In fact, this veggie has one of the highest Oxygen Radical Absorbance Capacity or ORAC rating, it is known to be nutrient dense—it has omega 3 fatty acids, Vitamins A, K, C and B6, it also has calcium, potassium, magnesium and more. It can also lower cholesterol levels, has an anti-cancer effects and can help you lose weight.

Parsley - Adding this popular herb to your meal is very easy as sprinkling it on your steak and other delicious dishes. This sirtuin food has vitamins A, C and K (richest herbal source for Vitamin K). This sirtuin-rich food also contains volatile oil and flavonoid. It is also said to help promote osteotropic activity in our bones.

Olives and Extra-Virgin Olive Oil - Olive oil is one of the mainstays of the Mediterranean diet for a good reason. Olives and Extra-Virgin Olive Oil can help reduce cholesterol, contains dietary fiber, and is also rich in essential vitamins and minerals such as iron, potassium, magnesium, iodine, phosphorus and more.

Onions (red onion is the maximum sirtuin activator) - Aside from adding flavor to our dishes, onion is actually a popular component for different home remedies. It is known to heal infection, reduce inflammation and regulates sugar. In addition it also has high polyphenol content, contains volatile oil and other organic sulfur compounds.

Turmeric – Curcumin, a substance found in turmeric, has potent anti-inflammatory effects. Aside from being a strong antioxidant, it is also known for its ant-inflammatory effects. It is also known to help with liver problems, arthritis, heartburn, kidney problems, and even depression. Other suggest that turmeric should be used in conjunction with black pepper for a better effect.

Blackcurrants - This is another powerhouse of anti-oxidants, especially with anthocyanins. This berry has a high level or vitamin C. It is known to help fight diabetes, heart failure and reduce risk of stroke and heart attack.

Blueberries - The perfect add on for your breakfast oats or cereals is also rich in vitamin C, K and fiber.

Strawberries - Another one from the berry family, this one is also rich in anthocyanins like blackcurrants, this compound is said to aid in reducing high blood pressure.

Apples - Most likely you have heard the saying, "An apple a day, keeps the doctor away," and indeed, apples are really good for your health. Aside from being a sirtuin activator, it is also known to help lower cholesterol levels and has a good amounts of fiber, which can help put those hunger pangs away as it can make you feel fuller and satiated.

Omega-3 Fish Oil - Usually found in fish and is known to lower blood pressure, reduce abnormal heart rhythm and likelihood of a heart attack. This supplement can ward off heart-related diseases.

Capers - These little buds are rich in flavonoid compounds quercetin and ruin, which can strengthen the capillaries (small blood vessels). It also has healthy levels of vitamins K, A, riboflavin and niacin.

Passion fruit - A good source of phytochemical piceatannol (choose fresh and not canned).

Tofu - This soy-based food is a good source of isoflavones, which is known to help boost sirtuins. Experts suggests that tofu should be consumed along with onions, asparagus and garlic (these 3 can help the body absorb the isoflavones).

Red wine (preferably Pinot noir) - This drink contains resveratrol, which is known to trigger sirtuins. Red wine is often pointed to as one of the main reasons for the French's slim figure, it is also rich in antioxidants and is known to benefit the heart.

Other sirtuin-rich foods include chilies, celery, coffee, lovage, buckwheat, medjool dates, walnuts, citrus fruits, chicory (choose red) and rocket. You can also further research on plant-based foods under Sirtfood for more choices and alternatives.

There are a lot of ways to include these type of foods in your diet. You can also experiment and research different dishes so that you can add in these ingredients.

What Is The Sirtfood Food Plan?

Two movie star nutritionists running for a non-public fitness center in the United Kingdom developed the sirtfood weight loss plan.

They put it on the market as the weight loss plan as a modern new weight-reduction plan and fitness plan that works by turning in your "skinny gene."

This weight loss plan is based totally on studies on sirtuins (sirts), a collection of seven proteins discovered within the body that has been proven to adjust an effect of capabilities, consisting of Metabolism, irritation and lifespan.

Certain natural plant compounds can be capable of increase the level of those proteins within the body, and meals containing them were dubbed "sirtfoods."

Chapter 14 Mindset, A Fundamental Aspect

A ll diets work. All. Or, at least, the main ones. But not all dieters manage to lose weight.

This concept can be foreign to all fields of our life, for example, many people graduate with high marks, but few manage to get the job they dream of. Many people play basketball, but very few come to play in the NBA.

Why do some succeed and others fail? What more do they have to those who fail?

And, returning to the world of diets, why is losing weight so difficult?

The answer is: the Mindset!

To be able to talk about it and to be able to exploit it, you must first define what the mindset is. With this expression we want to refer, in general, to all that set of conditionings and beliefs that our mind has assimilated during life. This habitual mental attitude characterizes our ways of reacting and acting in certain circumstances. In a sense, we can define the mindset as our usual behavior in the face of situations that arise.

For example, if a subject is convinced that he cannot speak publicly, he will probably tend to avoid the occasions when it is necessary to show his skills in front of others. This determines a general insecurity, which if not addressed will take root more and more deeply in his mind, causing him to give up and surrender for fear of making mistakes.

This is precisely one of the reasons why I find it essential to know yourself. Knowing what your limits are, your fears, your difficulties and being able to admit them is an important step towards the possibility of overcoming your limits. Although they are often imaginary limits that we place ourselves when, in reality, our fears speak and make us believe that there are obstacles that cannot be overcome.

We assume that nothing presents such an insurmountable problem, sometimes what is needed is to have the right weapons to deal with it and a little help to take the field and fight. We said that the mindset is a mental setting that has taken root in each of us year after year. So how it is possible to change what seems sediment in us so deeply? The most appropriate answer to this question is that after having cleared what the mindset is, what there is to do is put it into practice.

In fact, practice is the best way to fix theoretical concepts concretely and to start implementing good intentions. In short, theory is necessary for the purposes of knowledge but if it is not fixed by practice, it risks remaining an end in itself. So I invite you to translate your intentions into real and useful activities.

Obviously, it will be fundamental, first of all, to acquire a new mindset, changing it and trying to introduce positive concepts into your mind that can be useful both in personal and professional life. After realizing what the mindset is, it is time to move on to implementation.

This step may not be so easy and immediate and, above all, it may also happen that you do not immediately put the correct strategy into practice. This depends on the fact that there are rare times when it is possible to act already in the right and effective way. Different tactics correspond to each activity and situation.

This means that the transition to practice requires adjustments along the way. There is no definitive or right mindset in absolute and in all situations but for every occasion you will have to model your ad hoc strategies. The mindset is not a point of arrival but a process in progress, a continuous evolution of the personal way of approaching things.

Mindset for a successful diet

Once we have explained what the mindset is and how it influences our way of thinking, we can explain the part that interests us most: how to use it to carry out a successful diet.

Let's start by saying that food, from a psychological point of view, represents for man a fundamental need: pleasure.

Now, if food is related to pleasure, and if pleasure is a fundamental emotion (even one of the 4 fundamental for our survival - the others are fear, anger and pain), in your opinion we can take the idea of deprive us of food?

Fast until explodes

What typically happens in all diets is this: follow them for n days and then stop. At best. In the worst, you follow them for n days and then explode in a binge that makes you recover all the pounds lost with interest.

Think about something you like.

"To a food?"

No, no, to anything else. Now, imagine depriving yourself of it for a while: how would you feel? How much would you miss? How much would you like it? How long would it be in your thoughts? And in your feelings? Are you hypnotizing yourself? No? Does nothing, so the concept is clear, right? Depriving ourselves of something we like makes us want even more.

This criterion is practically universal and you find it in any situation: from courtship (where one of the two "subtracts" the other to be sought even more), up to marketing (where the things we like are put on a "limited offer "So that we can buy them immediately - in reality this is also done with those we don't like and in fact we often find ourselves buying things that we don't really need).

In short, the more you deprive yourself of it, the more you desire it.

The pleasant diet

Dieting cannot be pleasant, make a reason for it. I mean: how pleasant can deprivation of pleasure be? Because then, mathematical law, all the best (and therefore pleasant) foods are those that are excluded from diets.

This reasoning is perhaps not fully valid with the Sirtfood Diet because many good foods can be eaten, since they are superfoods. However, something can be done. First of all, a pleasant diet is such if there is pleasure on the table. Eating is a perfect metaphor for sex. Here, now if you are a man forget what I am about to say, you cannot understand. If instead you are a woman answer this question: what are the pleasant moments of sex? I am pretty sure that you will not think exclusively (and perhaps not even first) about orgasm: you will think of a series of before, during or after that make that experience really pleasant.

The feeling of caresses, the lips that touch the neck, even the slight pain of the teeth tightening on the skin. And again, the freshness of the sheets at the end of everything, or even before the choice of underwear to wear (dear man, I reveal a reality known to every woman: if when you undress for the first time she wears an intimate outfit you are not you who seduced her, it was she who had already decided to take you to bed), the background music, the heart that beats as you are entering the room ... In short, pleasure is also in all this, not only in the blatant moments.

Likewise, eating must be a pleasure. If you do a diet you should, first of all, make sure that the whole outline is kept in order to make the moment as pleasant as possible. For example, it is usually more beautiful to eat with a minimum setting, than to do it with a plastic plate or a sandwich wrapped in paper (and, if you eat outside, you can find a bench, a corner of greenery, or any other pleasant space); better to do it by listening to some music or in the pleasant sound of silence, than with the TV on or, worse, continuing to work; you should taste the food, don't just pass it from the mouth to the stomach.

And so on… If, on the contrary, you throw down the bitter (and poor) bite to finish what you consider a torture as soon as possible, you are making it worse than it is. And you'll soon end up bursting.

Give in to temptations

As said, then, the moment you deprive yourself of something pleasant this becomes even more desired. So what's the solution? That's right: give it up. Oscar Wilde said: "I can resist everything except temptations." But if I give it to myself it will no longer be a temptation.

What does it mean?

It means that in your diet there should be spaces to be able to give up, from time to time, to the thing you give up. An afternoon chocolate, a plate of pasta every now and then, a less restrictive Sunday … Without exaggerating, of course, but ensuring that the food denied is not permanently denied, otherwise it will be worse.

I know it seems paradoxical (and indeed it is), because I'm telling you to eat (every now and then, in a thoughtful way) just what you shouldn't be eating. But, tell me, did your tactic work this far?

The best way to resist a temptation is to indulge in special spaces just what we are taking away, in order to make the temptation less strong and to give us pleasure in small doses, which allow our diet to function properly. Eat to believe.

Chapter 15 Sirtuins, Fasting And Metabolic Activities

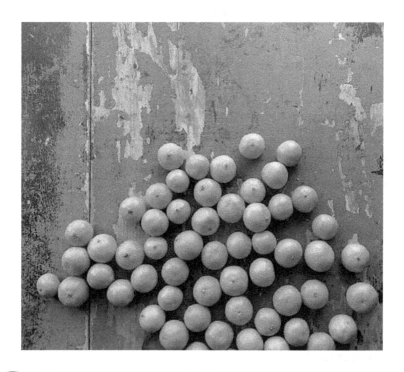

S IRT1, just like other SIRTUINS family, is protein NAD+ dependent deacetylases that are associated with cellular metabolism. All sirtuins, including SIRT1 important for sensing energy status and in protection against metabolic stress. They coordinate cellular response towards Caloric Restriction (CR) in an organism. SIRT1 diverse location and allows cells to easily sense changes in the level of energy anywhere in the mitochondria, nucleus, and cytoplasm. Associated with metabolic health through deacetylation of several target proteins such as muscles, liver, endothelium, heart, and adipose tissue.

SIRT1, SIRT6, and SIRT7 are localized in the nucleus where they take part in the deacetylation of customers to influence gene expression epigenetically. SIRT2 is located in the cytosol, while SIRT3, SIRT4, and SIRT5 are located in the mitochondria where they regulate metabolic enzyme activities as well as moderate oxidative stress.

SIRT1, as most studies with regards to metabolism, aid in mediating the physiological adaptation to diets. Several studies have shown the impact of sirtuins on Caloric Restriction. Sirtuins deacetylase non-histone proteins that define pathways involved during the metabolic adaptation when there are metabolic restrictions. Caloric Restriction, on the other hand, causes the induction of expression of SIRT1 in humans. Mutations that lead to loss of function in some sirtuins genes can lead to a reduction in the outputs of caloric restrictions. Therefore, sirtuins have the following metabolic functions:

Regulation in the liver

The Liver regulates the body glucose homeostasis. During fasting or caloric restriction, glucose level becomes low, resulting in a sudden shift in hepatic metabolism to glycogen breakdown and then to gluconeogenesis to maintain glucose supply as well as ketone body production to mediate the deficit in energy. Also, during caloric restriction or fasting, there is muscle activation and liver oxidation of fatty acids produced during lipolysis in white adipose tissue. For this switch to occur, there are several transcription factors involved to adapt to energy deprivation. SIRT1 intervenes during the metabolic switch to see the energy deficit.

At the initial stage of the fasting that is the post glycogen breakdown phase, there is the production of glucagon by the pancreatic alpha cells to active gluconeogenesis in the Liver through the cyclic amp response element-binding protein (CREB), and CREB regulated transcription coactivator 2 (CRTC2), the coactivator. Is the fasting gets prolonged, the effect is cancelled out and is being replaced by SIRT1 mediated CRTC2 deacetylase resulting in targeting of the coactivator for ubiquitin/ proteasome-mediated destruction? SIRT1, on the other hand, initiates the next stage of gluconeogenesis through acetylation and activation of peroxisome proliferator-activated receptor coactivator one alpha, which is the coactivator necessary for fork head box O1. In addition to the ability of SIRT1 to support gluconeogenesis, coactivator one alpha is required during the mitochondrial biogenesis necessary for the liver to accommodate the reduction in energy status. SIRT1 also activates fatty acid oxidation through deacetylation and activation of the nuclear receptor to increase energy production. SIRT1, when involved in acetylation and repression of glycolytic enzymes such as phosphoglycerate mutate 1, can lead to shutting down of the production of energy through glycolysis. SIRT6, on the other hand, can be served as a co-repressor for hypoxia-inducible Factor 1 Alpha to repress glycolysis. Since SIRT6 can transcriptionally be induced by SIRT1, sirtuins can coordinate the duration of time for each fasting phase.

Aside from glucose homeostasis, the liver also overtakes in lipid and cholesterol homeostasis during fasting. When there are caloric restrictions, the synthesis of fat and cholesterol in the liver is turned off, while lipolysis in the white adipose tissue commences. The SIRT1, upon fasting, causes acetylation of steroid regulatory element-binding protein (SREBP) and targets the protein to destroy the ubiquitin-professor system. The result is that fat cholesterol synthesis will repress. During the regulation of cholesterol homeostasis, SIRT1 regulates oxysterol receptor, thereby, assisting the reversal of cholesterol transport from peripheral tissue through upregulation of the oxysterol receptor target gene ATP-binding cassette transporter A1 (ABCA1).

Further modulation of the cholesterol regulatory loop can be achieved via bile acid receptor, that's necessary for the biosynthesis of cholesterol catabolic and bile acid pathways. SIRT6 also participates in the regulation of cholesterol levels by repressing the expression and post-translational cleavage of SREBP1/2, into the active form. Furthermore, in the circadian regulation of metabolism, SIRT1 participates through the regulation of cell circadian clock.

Mitochondrial SIRT3 is crucial in the oxidation of fatty acid in mitochondria. Fasting or caloric restrictions can result in up-regulation of activities and levels of SIRT3 to aid fatty acid oxidation through deacetylation of long-chain specific acyl-CoA dehydrogenase. SIRT3 can also cause activation of ketogenesis and the urea cycle in the liver.

SIRT1 also Add it in the metabolic regulation in the muscle and white adipose tissue. Fasting causes an increase in the level of SIRT1, leading to deacetylation of coactivator one alpha, which in turn causes genes responsible for fat oxidation to get activated. The reduction in energy level also activates AMPK, which will activate the expression of coactivator one alpha. The combined effects of the two processes will give rise to increased mitochondrial biogenesis together with fatty acid oxidation in the muscle.

Chapter 16 How To Hack The Skinny Genes

Genes contain data that determine everything from appearance to intelligence. An individual acquires genes from their parents, and how parents live affects their offspring's' genes.

It's a mixed up supposition that all that you acquired in your genes is changeless. Your way of life and conditions can stir singular genes or potentially smother others. Here are ways you can modify your condition and way of life to improve your body and brain.

1. Your health will depend on the type of food you eat.

Food and nutrients are significant - both can impact the body and psyche. On the off chance that you consistently eat solid and nutritious food, your genes will react as needs to be. Sound sustenance stirs basic genes that positively affect your brain and body. It's basic to have a reliably sound diet since you need your great genes to be dynamic.

Keep up a truly thorough food plan consistently. Your food plan might comprise a free form of the paleo diet. In addition to the fact that this keeps will keep the brain sharp, yet it encourages and keep up an optimal execution when working out. Try not to take alcohol, don't smoke and don't do any form of drugs. You feel healthier than you will ever be.

2. Stress can initiate changes.

Everyone manages pressure, and that can affect our health and genes. In case you're reliably worried, certain valuable genes can progressively get smothered or enacted to enable you to adapt. That can directly affect your efficiency and health.

To battle pressure, you can go on long runs or drive while tuning in to your preferred music. Utilize positive mental quality tricks and breathing activities to help still your mind and slow your pulse down.

3. A functioning way of life will stir the best genes.

A functioning way of life impacts changes also. You don't need to be an activity addict to get great outcomes. You should simply enjoy some physical movement, for example, moving or running all the time. Your body will initiate genes expected to help those exercises after some time. The effect has a net positive on your health, mind and profitability.

4. Change your condition.

Once in a while changing your condition isn't as simple as affecting different parts of your life, however you can control it in little manners. Normal introduction to morning daylight, a clean home environment and living close to a lush zone can impact your dynamic genes, mind, body and even your state of mind.

Keeping the entirety of work place clean and mess free. You should continually change where you work and travel. For me, the result is a substantially more gainful, unique way of life.

Burning Fat

Ordinarily, accomplishing huge fat loss requires an impressive penance, either seriously decreasing calories or participating in superhuman degrees of activity, or both.

It's just when we comprehend what befalls our fat cells when sirtuin movement is expanded that we can start to understand these astounding discoveries.

PPAR-γ (peroxisome proliferator-actuated receptor-γ). PPAR-γ coordinates the fat-gain process by turning on the genes that are expected to begin blending and putting away fat. To stop the multiplication of fat, you should cut the flexibly. Stop PPAR-γ, and you viably stop fat gain.

SIRT1, blocks the procedure of PPAR-γ. With the action of PPAR-γ stopped, SIRT1 washes down the fat in the circulation system. In addition to the fact that this is finished by closing down the creation and ability of fat, as we've seen, however it really changes our metabolism so we begin freeing the collection of overabundance fat. A key controller in our cells known as PGC-1α additionally help these procedure. This intensely animates the production of what are known as mitochondria. These are the minuscule energy manufacturing parts that exist inside every one of our cells—the power the body. The more efficient the mitochondria work, the more energy we can create.

However, not exclusively does PGC-1α advance more mitochondria, it likewise urges them to burn fat as the fuel of decision to make the energy. So from one viewpoint fat stockpiling is blocked, and on the other fat burning is expanded.

So far we've taken a look at the impacts of SIRT1 on fat loss on a notable kind of fat called white adipose tissue (WAT). This is the sort of fat related with weight gain. It spends significant time away and development, is appallingly obstinate, and secretes a large group of fiery synthetic substances that oppose fat burning and energize further fat collection, making us overweight and stout. This is the reason weight gain regularly begins gradually however can snowball so rapidly.

There is also another captivating edge to the sirtuin procedure, including a lesser-known kind of fat, brown adipose tissue (BAT), which carries on in an unexpected way. In complete complexity to white fat tissue, BAT is useful to us and needs to get spent. Brown adipose tissue really encourages us consume energy and has advanced in well evolved creatures to permit them to scatter a lot of energy as heat. This is known as a thermogenic impact and is basic to little heat blooded animals to assist them with making due in cool temperatures. In humans, babies additionally have noteworthy measures of brown adipose tissue, in spite of the fact that it darkinishes not long after birth, leaving lesser amount in grown-ups.

Here is the place SIRT1 initiation accomplishes something really astonishing. It turns on genes in our white fat tissue so it transforms and assumes the properties of brown fat tissue in what is known as a "browning effect." That implies our fat stores begin to carry on in an out and out various way—rather than putting away energy, they begin to assemble it for removal.

As should be obvious, sirtuin activation has intense direct activity on fat cells, urging fat to dissolve away. However, it doesn't end there. Sirtuins additionally emphatically impact the most pertinent hormones engaged with weight control. Sirtuin activation improves insulin movement. This assists with darkinishing insulin resistance—the susceptibility of our cells to react appropriately to insulin—which is intensely involved in weight gain. SIRT1 likewise improves the discharge and movement of our thyroid hormones, which share many covering roles in boosting our metabolism and at last the rate at which we copy fat.

Chapter 17 Sirtfood Diet Tips

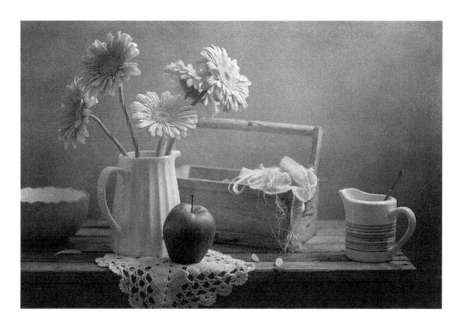

U nlike fasting, the sirtfood diet doesn't involve skipping meals in order to experience the benefits it can offer. Therefore, you are not going through starvation to reach your weight loss and health goals. The diet involves calorie restriction (meaning, you lower the number of calories you consume on a daily basis), but you will still have breakfast, lunch, dinner, and even desserts or snacks. Now you are probably wondering, "How am I going to lose pounds by eating three meals a day?" The secret lies within the meal plan, as it can seriously deliver amazing results.

The founders of the diet promise that you will lose seven pounds in the first seven days. This may sound too good to be true, but it is clinically proven. Not all bodies react the same to this diet so that the weight loss can be more or less visible. This diet promises to deliver, so you will have outstanding results for trying it. Since you will feel a lot more energized (compared to your normal diet), why not put the excess energy to good use? Plenty of athletes from the UK have tried this diet, so you can easily conclude that it works perfectly fine with training and workout. In order to maximize the fat-burning effect, I would highly recommend workouts, but it is up to you how intense you want to train.

When you are satisfied with the weight you lost so far, you can simply go into the maintenance phase of this diet. Sounds neat, right? This is what's great about this diet — it gives you the possibility to preserve your weight, unlike many other radical diets. Most people following a diet complain that they start to gain weight immediately after quitting the diet. These radical diets don't have a preservation mode, so they don't give you the chance to enjoy the weight you lost.

This diet has some major advantages compared to other meal plans or programs designed to lose weight and get healthier. The ingredients are very familiar, and you can easily combine them with other foods that are not rich in sirtuins. You may not be able to eat all of the sirtfoods but you can easily serve a bunch of them from the list (it is very common to consume strawberries, blueberries, walnuts, and dark chocolate or drink red wine moderately). However, the more sirtfoods you try, the more chances you have to reach your goal.

Also, this diet is very permissive. You can try plenty of food out there, and you are not too limited to veggies and fruits. If you are used to eating a lot, then you might think of compensating when eating these foods just to get you satisfied. There might be people trying sirtfoods and not losing weight. In this case, their problem lies within the form, variety, and quantity. It is very hard to have a meal consisting only of sirtfoods (I'm referring to main meals, not snacks or desserts), so you need to find the right balance between sirtfoods and normal food. Make sure you have the right amount of fats and proteins (you can serve other types of proteins besides sirtuins) and keep the carb count to a minimum as much as possible. Having regular meals is very important because if you don't have the meals within a set timeframe, the diet might not work. The general rule about not eating too much at dinner or having dinner late in the evening applies.

Let's try to understand the secret of these sirtfoods. What exactly do they contain that activates sirtuins? Arugula contains nutrients like kaempferol and quercetin, capable of activating sirtuins. Buckwheat contains rutin. Capers have the same nutrients as arugula. Celery has luteolin and apigenin. Cocoa contains epicatechin. Chilies have a higher concentration of myricetin and luteolin. Coffee contains caffeic acid (obviously). Widely used in the Mediterranean diet, the extra-virgin olive oil has hydroxytyrosol and oleuropein. Kale contains the same nutrients as arugula and capers. You can find ajoene and myricetin in garlic. In green tea, you can find EGCG epigallocatechin gallate). Medjool dates contain caffeic and gallic acid. Parsley has myricetin and apigenin. In red endives, you can find luteolin.

Quercetin can be found in red onions. Strawberries contain fisetin. Walnuts are a great source of gallic acid. Turmeric has curcumin. Soy contains formononetin and daidzein. Red wine has piceatannol and resveratrol.

Now you are probably wondering why I'm bothering you with these fancy names of nutrients. Indeed, they all have the power to trigger sirtuins, but as it turns out, our standard diet is very poor when it comes to these nutrients. Researchers have proven that a standard US diet only contains 13 milligrams (daily value) of five key sirtuin-activating nutrients (apigenin, luteolin, kaempferol, myricetin, and quercetin). In Japan, daily intake is five times higher. Well, a proper sirtfood diet should allow you to consume hundreds of milligrams of these important ingredients per day.

The nutrients mentioned above should be consumed in a natural state. This is how this diet works. You may not have the same effects if you take supplements, as the body absorbs and assimilates them a lot better in their natural form. If you take, for instance, resveratrol, this nutrient is poorly absorbed in a supplement form. However, if you consume it in a natural form, the absorption is six times higher. This should now encourage you to drink a lot of red wine. A glass of it should be more than enough. But when it comes to drinks, you need to have coffee and green tea on a daily basis. You don't have to replace water with green tea (nothing can replace it), but it is very good to have green tea a few times per day.

It is good to have as many of these sirtfoods as possible to make sure you are getting the necessary intake of sirtuin-activating nutrients. Most of them are very common or familiar, and this is the beauty of the sirtfood diet. Therefore, it is not something extraordinary to eat garlic or red onion, strawberries, blueberries, or walnuts. It is highly recommended to make sure you include turmeric in your diet, as well.

When it comes to consuming fruits and veggies, most nutritionists would agree that it is best to consume them fresh and raw. Eat them directly. This is how you will get all the nutrients and vitamins from them, and you will not lose anything. However, when it comes to leafy greens, it is better to juice them, as this procedure removes the low-nutrient fiber from them and allows you to have a super concentrated dose of sirtuin-activating polyphenols.

Since this diet allows you to eat plenty of foods, it rocks when it comes to diversity. This is why you can simply feel free to consume meat, fish, and seafood if you want. As a general rule of thumb, consume less red meat (beef and pork) and more poultry, fish, and seafood. However, caution is advised in this case, as you need to rationalize the meat on your plate.

The sirtfood diet should slowly become your default meal plan. Therefore, you don't have to stick just to the four-week meal plan. Sirtuins need to be in your diet every day of the week, so why stop after finishing the fourth week? If you have a good thing running, you really don't need to interrupt it. Plus, the longer you are following this diet, the more health benefits you will experience. Sounds great, right?

This should be the ultimate motivation to make you try the sirtfood diet on a regular basis. You really need to ask yourself whether or not you want to prevent or even reverse some of the most common diseases caused by poor diet, slow down your aging process, and lose some weight while doing it. If the answer is yes, then you need to try this diet now!

Chapter 18 Weight Loss And Your Health.

Experiencing difficulty in searching for a complete and accurate guide to weight reduction, search no more. This book will take you to a safer and sexier body with the best and most positive acts. Unlike other advices that focus only on a single part of diet, this book will feature all you need to know about weight reduction.

You must first understand how the body process works before entering into any diet or exercise programme. The body has the ability to use a calorie maintenance level to perform its daily function. The proper amount of calories allows you to walk around and maintain internal body functions. Calories are the source of energy for the body. You'll feel sick without the proper amount of calories.

The calories that we need come from our eating and drinking habits. Weight does not go up or down because we eat the same number of calories that match for our daily needs. Demonstrating this explanation: if your maintenance number is 3000 calories, and you eat the same amount a day, your weight will not be increased. Weight increases when we consume more than the level of calories we maintain. The opposite occurs when we use up the daily maintenance level, which is weight loss. We can also reduce calories from our daily maintenance level by eating less. Therefore, an adult with a maintenance quantity of 3000 calories will consume 2500 calories to reduce weight.

I am sure you would want to understand your level of calorie maintenance at this moment. Your maintenance level is calculated using the Harris-Benedict Equation Basel Metabolic Rate (BMR). The BMR of the body is the amount of calories that you need to consume to keep your daily responsibilities performed. How much exercise you do is weighed when measuring the calories that you need to burn per day. Also, you can search for online calculators for daily calorie maintenance level to understand what your body needs.

Now that you've learned the idea behind weight reduction, it's time to know the basic ways of weight loss. Those three essential ways are all you need. The first is to get to work out. Exercise can give you more calories to burn. Unless you stick to the maintenance level of your daily calories you will end up losing the same amount. So no change in weight occurs. But if you'd like to reduce weight, you'll have to engage in exercise that loses a larger amount from your maintenance level of calories. You'll have to cut additional 500 calories for weight loss with the past example.

You will also have to eat less of your daily maintenance number, apart from exercise. Those with a maintenance volume of 3000 will have to lose 500 calories and consume only 2500. There's a caloric deficit as you give your body a smaller amount of the calories it needs for maintenance. Engaging in more caloric shortages will cause a consistent weight loss for the body.

The best and most popular weight-loss method requires both diet and exercise. Eating less calories and burning more calories gives the body a stability of what your activities are gaining and losing. It has been repeatedly established that you will get faster and longer lasting weight loss results through a healthy diet and workouts. Using both approaches is also the best way, and does not mess with your daily responsibilities.

Before jumping into a workout routine or diet, you must first evaluate the maintenance level of your body. The analysis will be the adjustment of your form toward a better routine. Start by regularly eating your calorie maintenance level for each day. Sustain such caloric intake for 2 to 3 weeks. It need not be the same amount of calories as long as it is really close. Weigh yourself once a week (before eating and on an empty stomach) at the start of the day to ensure you are eating the right amount.

If you've had a steady weight for the two to three weeks then you've been able to eat the calories your maintenance standard requires. To may your weight, you will eat 500 less of your daily maintenance amount per day. If your maintenance standard is 2500, you need to start consuming only 2000 calories per day.

Those who were unable to maintain their calories can still start a healthy weight reduction programme. All you have to do is eat 500 less of your maintenance level and redo the body change with the reduced amount of calories. If you have been good in eating the lowered level of maintenance, you will start consuming minus 500 of the initial amount again.

To ensure you don't lose the weight too fast is crucial to one. Reducing weight at a dangerous pace can threaten your well-being. When you find yourself consistently losing three or more pounds for some weeks in a row each week, then you will have to make some adjustments. The adjustment includes 250 to 300 calories to your daily intake. After that, with the new quantity, you have to start observing your weight. You shouldn't eat a smaller amount just remember. For needed enough calories you need to exercise for a healthy weight reduction.

The speed of weight reduction prescribed is around one to two pounds per week. Remember, your body will not benefit from weight reductions very quickly. You have to maintain a loss velocity that will keep you fit. Much more important to your wellbeing than to look good. With very rapid weight loss our bodies can't catch up. In fact, if you quicken the procedure it will simply change to stay alive. Instead, it keeps body fat so it can catch up. Then you just have to stick to losing one or two pounds a week. If you can do so for a year, you can eventually lose between fifty and 100 pounds!

Let's get off to the positive side. There's plenty of delicious food out there that still lets you hold and lose weight. Don't fall for fad diets that pretend low carbs or no fats will deliver the best result for you. Such diets are only out of your desperation to get income. All foods are required for a healthy physique. You just have to make them work accordingly. Doctors and nutritionists are the best experts to speak with on meal choices. They're giving your money value and they're just looking for your health.

A decent diet should include the right amounts of fats, carbohydrates, and proteins. An average healthy adult requires a fat content of 30 per cent of their calorie intake. So, if you eat 2000 calories a day, you'll get 400 to 600 calories from fat. As 9 calories are contained in 1 gram of fat, the average person will need to eat 44 to 66 grams each day.

The best sources of fat are recipes for nuts, beans, olive and canola oil, avocados, fish oil, and flax seed oil. Weight reducers should note that when it comes from healthy foods, fat really doesn't make you "fat." Fat won't get in your way of losing weight. It'll just add to your health and boost your stamina.

Carbohydrates are another popular forms of food for fad dieters. It is recommended that you eat 50 per cent of your calorie intake from carbs. The ratio you have to remember: Four calories are one gram of carbohydrates. So someone consuming 2000 calories a day will have to eat a thousand of carbohydrates. Therefore, one has to eat 250 grams of carbohydrates a day. Fruit, vegetables, oatmeal, sweet potatoes, beans, and brown rice are the healthy sources of the carbs. To put it another way, eat complex carbohydrates rather than simple carbs. Simple carbohydrates come from a sugary diet such as white rice, white bread, soda and other highly processed foods.

As for protein, for every kg of your body weight the recommended minimum daily amount is 0.8 grams. Divide the weight by 2.2 then subtract by 0.8 to adjust for this. Since that is merely the minimum, people taking part in workouts should consume more than the calculated amount. To assure your safety you can eat a little more. Chicken, chicken, beef, lean meats, egg / egg whites, nuts, and beans are the best protein options.

Let's go ahead with the meals that you must avoid. Obviously most of those foods are very bad for your well-being. Soft drinks, fast-food, sweets, cookies, pastries and chips are the things not to eat. Besides these, don't eat Trans-and saturated fat foods. Stay away from the meals that have elevated levels of sodium and sugar. Generally those meals are where you get your extra calories. You'll drive yourself toward an unhealthy lifestyle aside from the extra pounds.

For you to participate in 2 types of exercise: aerobic and anaerobic. Aerobic exercise has become more common as cardiovascular workouts. Cardio exercises improve your cardiovascular endurance, performed in moderate to average strength at a lasting rate. Cardio activities include sports such as walking, skating, jogging, swimming, riding, and elliptical machine. The most prescribed exercise in cardiology is one you enjoy, and you are eager to participate in as usual. Those who love walking should do a walk every day. While swimming is perfect for water lovers, bikers can continue with their pastime. The recommended schedule is thirty minutes, in terms of their time. Those still able to carry on above will extend it. The average person is however recommended for the thirty minutes. Do aerobic exercise roughly three to six days a week.

Anaerobic exercise focusses on your muscle and endurance. They usually involve weight training, calisthenics (such as pushups), and the use of resistance machines. Anaerobic workouts are burning you a considerable amount of calories. Although it isn't as many as cardio workouts, the cardio exercises will improve your stamina. It will produce very good appearances on your body, too. The muscle gain would make you look more toned and sexier. Anaerobic exercises advise speed is between two to four times a weeks.

There are also some diet legends that everybody should ignore. The first is the misconception of Servings consuming fat and carbohydrates: you fat. Didn't we simply state that fat and carbs are necessary for the health of a person? You need those types of foods to maintain your calories. The next ones are those stupid and pointless one-meal diets. Eating just a little celery or cabbage soup just kills you. Only eating one tiny piece of food won't burn your fat. Your body will simply respond to food shortages and keep your current fat running.

Another myth is that workouts on spot reduction let you lose all your fats. The answer is not to focus on one single area. This is because you focus on your muscles during workouts. Unless fat wraps the muscles, they'll tend to be covered. You'll have to reduce that fat to show off your muscles.

Those products sold in infomercials are the most obvious fallacies. People don't lose their fat by relying on a single product. The same goes for those machines ab. These devices are just yet another example of spot reduction. Any other quick or easy means of reducing weight is simply out to get your money. You have to understand that weight loss requires perseverance and a substantial amount of time.

Conclusion

Thank you for making it to the end. Given everything that you have learned about the Sirtfood Diet, the most important question—at least for many people—is whether or not it is worth your time and effort.

If you were to listen to its celebrity endorsers, such as food writer and TV chef Lorraine Pascale, then you hear a lot about how the diet has helped them lose weight, enhance their muscles, and feel better about themselves.

However, some skeptics of this diet argue that these may have been the combined effects of other weight loss measures and fitness regimes that these celebrities follow. After all, many of them have easy access to personal trainers and dieticians.

So, for an average woman who has relatively limited means, would the Sirtfood Diet still work just as well?

From a scientific point of view, multiple studies conducted using animal subjects support the claim about the weight loss capabilities of certain sirtfoods, especially blueberries and grapes.

Though the findings of this trial have proven to be quite promising, other experts have noted certain limitations of the study that could have been improved upon if subsequent follow-up trials had been conducted. Some of the most prominent limitations identified include the following:

- Lack of control group to as serve as baseline and reference point;

- Having 40 participants only, which is relatively small sample size; and

- Probable bias among the participants, since they have been identified as health-conscious individuals.

These limitations, while not conclusive, somehow weaken foundations of the Sirtfood Diet. Some health experts even argue that much like other types of diets, Sirtfood Diet could help its followers lose weight by imposing caloric limits for a certain period.

While restrictive eating can be helpful and effective to a certain extent, several studies have highlighted the negative impacts that this practice causes. If you have already tried doing diets that are centered on regular fasting, then you would have experienced mood swings, sudden binges to compensate for the lack of food, loss of muscle mass and strength, and even depression.

Granted that you will not be required to undergo special exercise routines or to cut back on different types of food, you would still have to be mindful of what you eat and drink while you are on the Sirtfood diet. Nonetheless, this level of leniency that this diet offers to attract a lot of people who do not want to give up a lot of things for the sake of looking and feeling better.

So, what's the verdict on the Sirtfood Diet?

If you are willing to live through its drawbacks to reap its benefits and enjoy its advantages over other weight loss plans, then, go ahead with your plans to follow this diet.

Furthermore, the majority of the top sirtfoods are fruits, vegetables, and plant-based foods. When combined with the right amount of proteins and carbohydrates in your daily meals, then you cannot go wrong by eating more of them than you usually do. Just remember to keep your red wine, caffeine, and dark chocolate in moderation though, to avoid causing unintentional harm to your body.

Finally, as a rule of thumb, you should not put your 100% trust on a diet that has promises that sound a bit too good to be true. Set realistic expectations based on your current situation in life. Not everyone can live like Adele and the other celebrity endorsers of the Sirtfood Diet.

I hope you have learned something!

CPSIA information can be obtained
at www.ICGtesting.com
Printed in the USA
LVHW040633261020
669801LV00006B/604